Meditations for Women Who Do Too Much

Other Books by Anne Wilson Schaef, Ph.D.

WOMEN'S REALITY

CO-DEPENDENCE MISUNDERSTOOD, MISTREATED

WHEN SOCIETY BECOMES AN ADDICT

THE ADDICTIVE ORGANIZATION (WITH DIANE FASSEL)

ESCAPE FROM INTIMACY

MEDITATIONS FOR LIVING IN BALANCE

Credits are listed following the index.

HarperCollins books may be purchased for educational, business, or sales promotional use. For information please write: Special Markets Department, HarperCollins Publishers, 10 East 53rd Street, New York, NY 10022.

HarperCollins Web site: http://www.harpercollins.com

HarperCollins®, 🏭 ®, and HarperOne™ are trademarks of HarperCollins Publishers.

Library of Congress Cataloging-in-Publication Data
Schaef, Anne Wilson.
    Meditations for women who do too much/Anne Wilson Schaef–[Rev. ed.].
    p. cm.
    Includes index.
    ISBN: 978–0–06–073624–8
    1. Women—prayer-books and devotions—English
    2. Devotional calendars. I.Title.
    BV4527.S27 2004
    158.1'28'082—dc22
                                                      2004054098

10 11 12 CW 20 19 18 17 16 15

✌ Introduction, 2004

It is with great pleasure that I introduce this new revised edition of *Meditations for Women Who Do Too Much*. The original book, published in 1990, was an instant success and sold over two million in the United States alone. That edition has been translated into many, many languages and has proved to be a bestseller throughout the world. It hit a nerve! If there is anything that women the world over have in common—crossing racial, religious, socioeconomic, and social lines—it is that we all do too much. We have been described as workaholics, careaholics, rushaholics, and busyaholics, and we are often so busy and distracted that we forget to take care of ourselves. Most of us would not describe ourselves as one of the "aholics" and almost all of us would agree that we quite simply do too much. Doing too much seems to be a given for most women.

How long have we known about this phenomenon? A long time. Florence Nightingale, who died in 1910, said, "Women never have a half-hour in all their lives (except before or after anybody is up in the house) that they can call their own, without fear of offending or of hurting someone. Why do people sit up so late, or, more rarely, get up so early? Not because the day is not long enough, but because they have no time in the day themselves."

In the eighties and nineties we talked about workaholism, careaholism (co-dependence and Al-Anon), rushaholism, and busyaholism, and some were helped by working a twelve-step program. We defined workaholism as the "addiction of choice of the 'unworthy.'" A little earlier (1960s and 1970s) women had tackled the subtle yet intense cultural brainwashing acculturation that had convinced us at a very deep, often unconscious level that we were, indeed, undeserving and unworthy in the eyes of the culture and suffered from "The Original Sin of Being Born Female" (discussed in *Women's Reality* [1981]). Some of us had hoped that after all that "consciousness raising" there would be major shifts in the way we women lived, worked, and thought of ourselves. Some changes have certainly occurred and we have shifted internally as women. Yet, as we moved into the jobs that men have traditionally held and into the new millennium, we were still doing too much. We had just added new professional responsibilities to the tasks women were already doing within a stepped-up society, where intensity and two-profession families are the norm not the exception. Even more is expected of us women, and we make great demands upon ourselves.

We have also developed some new labels to describe our lives. We now talk about "multi-tasking." Women have been multi-tasking for centuries, yet, with a new label one can be fooled into believing it is a new phenomenon. And the illusion of a "new phenomenon" allows us to deny the pressure of long-range, un-dealt-with problems. In fact, it would be interesting to speculate on the many repercussions of the phenomenon of renaming and making something that has traditionally been destructive a "new problem." Doing too much is not a new phenomenon *and* it continues to be a problem we women face every day. We are stretched thinner and thinner as we try to cope with our lives and make them productive, meaningful, and fun for ourselves and others.

Silicon Valley has generated a new acronym for the problem, BOSS (burnout stress syndrome), a problem it has even outsourced to India. Shauli Kaushik, 21, of India, who works at an India-based U.S. call center, says, "It's a tough life. It reduces life to a vacuum. Where's the time to lead a normal existence? I work hard but this is no life. I'm going to quit soon."

Current newspapers run articles on employers tightening down on "ease" in the workplace. Women no longer have time to run errands, go to the dentist, or take their children to doctor's appointments during work. Their employers want them "on the job" 100 percent of the time. The stress is increasing, and with it women are doing even more and taking care of themselves, their relationships, their health, their spirituality, and their creativity even less. There was a time in the not too distant past when some corporations were setting up "nap" rooms at the office, recognizing that in high-stress jobs some needed to lean back, rest, and "cool out" for a few minutes. Rest during the day was thought to increase productivity. Unfortunately, the "nap room phase" was short-lived.

While the labels describing the issue have changed, clearly the problem hasn't gone away. If anything, the problem has worsened.

I even wonder if women who do too much have time to read a meditation book anymore. One woman, a bank executive, told me that she keeps a copy of *Meditations for Women Who Do Too Much* in her desk, and when she feels particularly stressed she randomly opens it and reads a page. "It always helps," she says. "No matter what page it is it always seems to be just right for the moment. I don't have time to read it regularly." Perhaps we need to offer an online version so that many busy women can start their day with something "helpful." The yearly calendar for women who do too much does have an online component and from what I am told, it is used.

Many factors have convinced me that the issues addressed in this book are still relevant to today's women, perhaps even more so than before. So we decided to do a revision of *Meditations for Women Who Do Too Much,* not only to address the perennial issues women face but to address issues unique to the young women of today.

So many women have said to me, "I love the quotes. I didn't know about all these women and all this wisdom." Neither did I. In the process of writing both the original and this revision, I have met so many wise and powerful women! As Hillary Rodham Clinton has said, "One of my favorite times was reading quote books, which I did for hours on end." Me, too! The quotes are like a warm bath for many of us. We need to know that there have been wise women spreading wisdom throughout the ages and still are among us. What utter delight. We can utilize and build on that wisdom. We can make ages of women's wisdom our own.

As I read the quote books and researched for new, more contemporary material, I again became convinced that there are so many rich quotes and an abundance of new material. I was loving writing the new meditation pages. New quotes spurred new ideas. Contemporary women were continuing to share their humor and wisdom.

And thus we have this new revised edition, which mixes the old with the new. I realized from much feedback that some women are attached to certain "favorite" meditations in the original edition. If I have taken your favorite day out, I am sorry. Please write me through the publisher or at my address at the end of the Introduction and I guarantee it will be in the next book.

So, here it is—my best effort to update an old "classic."

This new edition will follow the same format as the original. There will be a quote, a meditation, information (reaction to the quote), and a short, reflective sentence for healing and moving on.

I have scattered completely new pages throughout the book. These have quotes from contemporary women (mostly—there are a few oldies but goodies I simply could not resist), and many new awarenesses about this business of doing too much and things we women might want to take note of as we cope with this modern life in the new millennium.

I have also left a few extra meditations in the back. I fully realize that not every meditation will be relevant to all women all of the time. Since we are strong and aware women who deserve choices (one of the essences of this book is to help us know that we have choices), I have made sure that we, indeed, have choices. So, look to the "extras" in the back if a single meditation just does not fit for you. Or, look to the extras in the back just for abundance.

These meditations do not tell you what to do, they do not tell you how you should be, and they are not answers. They are intended to stir up feelings, get you thinking, and precipitate possibilities for change that will add to the quality and vitality of your life. These meditations can be experienced as an open door, a direct hit to the solar plexus, comfort and companionship—or whatever. Make of them what you will.

I hope the book is helpful, enjoyable, meaningful, and, at times, challenging for you. It has been for me, and all of us deserve nothing less.

Enjoy! And let me know what you think. Write to me through my publisher or at my office, P.O. Box 990, Boulder, MT 59632–0990, or by email at wsa@gte.net.

Thank you for letting me become a part of your lives for a while.

Anne Wilson Schaef, Ph.D.

❧ January 1

RUSHING/FRENZY

Anything worth doing is worth doing frantically.

—New proverb

We women who do too much find the ending of an old year and the beginning of a new year to be a difficult time. There is always the temptation to try to "tidy up" all our loose ends as the old year closes. We fall into the trap of believing that it is possible to get our entire life "caught up" before starting a new year, and we are determined to do it.

Also, there is the temptation to set up an elaborate set of resolutions for the coming year so that we can, at last, *get it right*. As workaholics, we tend to be very hard on ourselves: nothing less than perfection is enough. Hopefully, on this first day of the year, we will be able to remember that we are perfect just as we are.

I HOPE for the willingness to live this year in a way that will be gentle to myself . . . one day at a time.

✣ January 2

COMMON SENSE

Did you ever stop to think that we women who do too much wouldn't be able to do too much if we weren't competent, strong, intelligent, courageous, and determined?

We might, however, be a bit lacking in common sense.

—Anne Wilson Schaef

We are powerful women with many skills. This is true even if we don't always feel so powerful or skillful. We have strong bodies, strong minds, and strong hearts that all serve us well—maybe too well. When we use the gifts we have been given and those we have so carefully worked to earn in destructive ways, maybe we have missed something in the "common sense" aspect of our skill-building.

Common sense is knowing when to quit. Common sense is knowing that we are good and not always having to prove it. Common sense is listening to those parts of our being that are put there to balance intelligence, competence, and determination. Common sense is rarely taught and is more likely observed. Common sense must be learned and is usually not genetic. Common sense is all too often discovered in old age and more useful when developed when we are younger.

Common sense gives us the ability to utilize our talents while staying in balance.

WHEN WE ADD **common sense to the mix, our other skills become more efficient and more constructive.**

❧ January 3

EXCUSES/CHOICES

So at an early age I witnessed the fact that work was of the first importance, and that it justified rather inhuman behavior.

—May Sarton

Workaholism, just like other addictions, is intergenerational. Many of us have learned it at home from our mothers and fathers, and we cannot even imagine any other way of being in this world. Work took precedence over everything in our households and families. We could only have fun after the work was done, and the work was never done. We could only relax and take care of our personal needs when the chores were completed and the house had been straightened up. And when that was done, we were much too tired to do anything else. Cleanliness was always next to godliness, and many times godliness seemed very far away.

Work was always tied to the necessities of life, getting ahead, and the American dream, and these ideals justified anything, even cruel and inhuman behavior in the family.

We learned our lessons well, and now we have the opportunity to break the intergenerational chain of workaholism. We have a chance to be different. We have choices.

LET ME NOTICE today how many times I use work as an excuse for my inhuman behavior.

HUMOR

Time wounds all heels.

—Jane Ace

We lose the ability to laugh *at* ourselves and *with* others.

Humor is so healing . . . and it's fun too. We find that humor is one of the first human gifts to disappear when we do too much.

We lose the ability to laugh *at* ourselves and *with* others. We feel insulted if someone pokes fun at us, and we personalize everything, seeing it as a put-down. The more our overworking takes over, the more we make Scrooge look like a stand-up comic. Indeed, instead of being heal*ers* we have become heels . . . heels without souls.

Good humor is very inexpensive. It is one of the pleasures in life that is relatively free. I'm sure, if we try hard enough, we can remember a part of us that used to laugh and be playful.

HUMOR **doesn't die, thank goodness, it just goes underground sometimes and digs caverns for our "serious" selves to cave in to.**

❧ January 5

CRISIS/EXHAUSTION/CONTROL

The sky is falling! The sky is falling!

—Chicken Little

Living our lives like Chicken Little can be quite exhausting. Yet so many of us live from one crisis to another! We have become so accustomed to crises and deadlines that we feel almost lost if we are not putting out some kind of fire. In fact, if we really were honest, there is something dramatic and exciting about handling a crisis. It makes us feel as if we have some modicum of control in our lives.

We have, however, on occasion wondered if all these crises are normal and if there is another way to live life that might be a little less exhausting. Even though we are exhilarated in handling these crises, they do leave us feeling drained. Could it be that these things don't just *happen* to us? That we have a hand in their creation?

As we begin to take a look, we see others around us who do not live from one crisis to another, and they seem to do just fine . . . they're even serene.

CRISIS and my illusion of control are not unrelated. I hope I will allow myself to be open to noticing the relationship between the two in my life today.

SELF-DECEPTION/ILLUSIONS

> *We live in a system built on illusions and when we put forth our own perceptions, we're told we don't understand reality. When reality is illusion and illusion is reality, it's no wonder we feel crazy.*
>
> —Anne Wilson Schaef

So much of our world is built on illusions. The illusion of control, the illusion of perfectionism, the illusion of objectivity. Dishonesty and denial are the building blocks of doing too much. When we participate in any of these illusions, we are deceiving ourselves, and when we deceive ourselves, we lose ourselves. Why is it that we find self-deception and illusions so much more attractive than honesty? It could possibly be because we are surrounded by a society where illusion is the name of the game. Denial runs rampant at every level of our society, and there is not much support for "truth speakers."

Yet, we are the only ones who can deceive ourselves. We are the only ones who can refuse to acknowledge our perceptions and lie to ourselves. The choice to deceive ourselves is ours.

THERE IS **an old saying, "Conscience is a cur that will let you get past it but that you cannot keep from barking." Sometimes our awareness makes funny noises to get our attention.**

RIGIDITY

> *Changes [in life] are not only possible and predictable,*
> *but to deny them is to be an accomplice to one's own*
> *unnecessary vegetation.*

—Gail Sheehy

Part of the crazy thinking we have developed is that we will be safe if we can just get everything in order, everything in place, and keep it that way. Much of our energy is spent trying to contribute to the calcification of our lives. Unfortunately, calcified beings are brittle and break easily.

When we become rigid about anything, we lose touch with our life process and place ourselves outside of the stream of life—we die. As Lillian Smith says, "when you stop learning, stop listening, stop looking and asking questions, always new questions, then it is time to die."

HAVE I already died? Am I one of the walking dead? Rigid isn't stable, it's just brittle.

✢ January 8

NEED TO ACHIEVE

Some of us are becoming the men we wanted to marry.
                                                    —Gloria Steinem

Getting an important position in a good company is an exacting feat. Many of us have worked long and hard to get where we are and we are proud of our achievements.

Success demands sacrifice and focus, and we have learned how to do both. We have put our work before everything else in our life. We have learned to compete and compromise. We have learned to dress like men and hold our own in a circle of men. We have learned to be tough and to "come on strong" when we need to. We wanted to make it in a man's world, and we have. We have learned to play the game.

It is time to stop and see what has happened to us in this process. Are we the *women* we want to be?

I WONDER if I have really become the man I would want to marry? Would my clear and healthy woman want to marry me?

ANGER

> *Anger as soon as fed is dead*
> *'Tis starving makes it fat.*

> —Emily Dickinson

Anger has not been an easy emotion for us. We get angry when we are passed over for promotions. We get angry when no one listens. We get angry when our ideas are not heard and even angrier when these same ideas are declared "fantastic" when one of our male colleagues presents them. We get angry when we are so strung out and exhausted that we find ourselves yelling at those we love the most. Then we become angry about being angry, and we try to "control ourselves."

It is important to remember that feelings are just that . . . feelings. It is normal for us to have feelings, and it is normal for us to feel anger. Anger is only harmful when it is held in and "starved" as Emily Dickinson says. When we hold it in, it builds and we find ourselves exploding on innocent people in the most astounding circumstances. Then we end up feeling bad about ourselves and getting anger backlash from others. We need to find safe places to let our anger out. We can respect our anger. It is our friend. It lets us know when something is wrong.

ANGER **is not the problem. What I do with it is.**

JUGGLING PROJECTS/NEGATIVISM

*I don't give myself credit for what I do get done because
I have so many projects hanging fire that I haven't done.*

—Chris

We workaholics are the type of people who see a glass half-empty instead of half-full. It is much easier to see what we haven't done than it is to see what we have done.

Often, if we just stop to take stock, we have really accomplished quite a bit. In fact, we probably have been a wee bit close to the edge of working wonders.

Unfortunately, we miss the opportunity to marvel at our wonders because we have so much set up still to do that what we have done pales into insignificance in relation to what is (always!) yet to be done. Ugly is in the eye of the beholder.

TODAY is awareness day for what I *have* accomplished. Celebrations may be in order.

❧ January 11

CHANGE/SECURITY

People change and forget to tell each other.
                                    —Lillian Hellman

How tenaciously we cling to the illusion that we will get our lives in order and they will stay that way! How resistant we are to the normal process of change! We often feel personally attacked if someone near and dear to us changes without clearing those changes with us first. We have somehow come to believe that security and stasis are synonymous.

Change is the manifestation of our ability to grow and become. When it occurs in those nearest and dearest to us it is an opportunity for celebration. When it happens in ourselves, it allows us to share ourselves on a new level. When we try to protect others from the awareness of our changes, we are being dishonest. No one can care for who we are unless they *know* who we are.

THE ONLY constant is change.

❧ January 12

MENOPAUSE

> *I believe menopause is a time when a woman's power, wisdom, and creativity pushes to the surface, calling for her attention.*
>
> —Christiane Northrup

Don't you think it's strange that "a time when a woman's power, wisdom, and creativity pushes to the surface, calling for her attention" has become a "medical problem" for which medication is required?

I remember when I "did" menopause. It was one of the "fiery" times of my life. I literally "glowed" with hot flashes. I also came to the conclusion that we women are not irritable during menopause because of hormones. We're irritable because of lack of sleep—on with the covers—off with the covers—on with the covers. . . . Those hot flashes kept me busy. Thank goodness they didn't last long.

I didn't fight it. I didn't resent it. I didn't see it as a disease, and it passed rather quickly. I did, surprisingly, at times, miss the "flushing" experience of my periods. The ultimate was when I married a much younger man and the first time we made love he conscientiously brought up the issue of birth control.

"No need," I said proudly.

"Aren't older women great?" he said, grinning.

WHO KNOWS what we'll do when our full power is unleashed. We may have to get younger men to keep up with us!

❧ January 13

COMPASSION/RUTHLESSNESS

> *And beyond even self-doubt no writer can justify ruthlessness for the sake of his work, because being human to the fullest possible extent is what his work demands of him.*
>
> —May Sarton

What May Sarton has written is not just true for a writer. No one can justify ruthlessness!

We are told that one has to be ruthless to make it in the world of business. As women, we have believed that we have to be even more ruthless than men just because we are women. Many of us have achieved success, but at what price? We don't like who we see in the mirror.

One of the characteristics of doing too much is that we progressively lose touch with our own morality and our own spirituality. We progressively lose touch with our humanness. We can, however, recover the possibility to reconnect with our compassionate self.

MY ABILITY to be compassionate and experience the beauty of my humanness has not left me. It was only buried under layers of garbage.

❧ January 14

BELIEF

> *Why indeed must "God" be a noun? Why not a verb . . .*
> *the most active and dynamic of all?*
>
> —Mary Daly

Some of us have difficulty with the concept of God because we have seen God evolve into something or someone who is static, a mega-controller, and frankly someone who is not that nice to be around. Traditionally, we have tried to make God static so we would feel safe. That is our problem, not God's.

What if we see God as a process—the process of the universe? What if we begin to understand that we are part of the process of the universe? What if we realize that it is only when we live who we are that we have the option of being one with that process? Trying to be someone else, who we *think* we should be or who *others* think we should be, ruptures our oneness with that process.

IF GOD is a process and I am a process, we have something in common with which to begin.

GIFTS

Make good use of bad rubbish.

—Elizabeth Beresford

It's really up to us what we do with our lives. We may have been battered, beaten, molested, incested, spoiled, or overindulged. All of us have feelings and memories we need to work through. None of us had perfect families. In fact, dysfunctional families are the norm for the society.

The question for us is how have our experiences affected us and what do we need to do to learn from our experiences, to work through those lessons, integrate them into our being, turn them over, and move on?

When we get stuck in our blame, anger, hurt, and denial, we are the ones who suffer. It is up to us to "make good use of bad rubbish."

IF MY LIFE resembles a garbage dump, it is up to me to sort it through, turn over the soil, and plant flowers to make use of all the natural fertilizer.

AMUSING GOD

> *God and I have a good relationship, but we both see other people.*

> —Dolly Parton

Often it occurs to me that God created human beings for amusement. And we certainly are a funny lot.

Often, as I sit in airports between flights, I avail myself of God's entertainment and just watch people. (I don't think God is selfish or protective about this entertainment. We are here for all of us to enjoy!)

For example, let's take denial. We can completely convince ourselves that we are not killing ourselves by doing too much, that we *have* to do too much, and that we have no other choices.

Now *that's* funny!

We thoroughly believe that we can hide our little "secrets" —over-buying, over-eating, over-doing . . . even affairs—and no one will be the wiser.

Aren't we a hoot?! We think that no one "sees" or "knows" our "secrets." We *are* a funny lot. We rush around pretending that no one knows our secrets and how they are affecting us when we are the only ones fooled. We are hysterically funny in our illusions. We *are* indeed entertaining.

IF GOD **created us for amusement and entertainment, we are doing a very good job.**

THINKING

> *To achieve, you need thought.... You have to know what you are doing and that's real power.*
>
> —Ayn Rand

Thinking sometimes takes a bum rap in some circles, and it is over-exaggerated in others! As a society, we have become so lopsided in rational, logical, and linear thinking that many of us have become confused about the process of thinking. We are very dualistic in our thinking about thinking.

We have come to believe that we must either be cold, calculating, logical, rational women, or we must throw all thinking out the window and carry the load for all the feeling, intuitive aspects of our society. Either of these solutions results in a languishing lopsidedness that leaves us wanting.

There is nothing wrong with thinking. It's the *way* we do it. Often, when we lead with our logical, rational minds, we have not allowed them to be informed by our being and our other thought processes of intuition, attention, and awareness. It is in the synergy among all these aspects of our mind that true thinking begins.

MY BRAIN is a great gift. Using all of it increases its value.

LIVING IN THE MOMENT

Love the moment, and the energy of that moment will spread beyond all boundaries.

—Corita Kent

We women who do too much have a terrible time loving the moment. We are always making lists and eyeing the tasks that are just around the corner when we need to be busy working on the task at hand. Hence, rarely does anything get our full, undivided attention. Because of this subtle distractibility and lack of presence, we miss a lot.

When we really can be in the moment, the very process of being in the moment radiates into the crevices of our life and begins to dust out the cobwebby corners.

PRESENCE is such a gift . . . to myself and others.

❧ January 19

CONTROL

People who try to boss themselves always want (however kindly) to boss other people. They always think they know best and are so stern and resolute about it they are not very open to new and better ideas.

—Brenda Ueland

We workaholics are difficult to be around. We are hard to work with and hard to work for. Our core form of functioning is control. We often do not know the difference between getting the job done and getting the job done well. Our belief is that if we can just control *everything*, we are doing our job and doing it right. Our illusion of control is killing us. We find ourselves exhausted and burned out.

Unfortunately, control is costly. In trying to realize this illusion of control, we are destructive to ourselves and others. Also, in trying to maintain this illusionary control, we find our field of vision becomes more and more constricted (as do our blood vessels!) and we are no longer open to new and better ideas. In fact we are not open to any ideas at all.

WHEN, in my controlling behavior, I do unto others as I do unto myself, we all lose.

❧ January 20

CONTROL

> *She was a "what if" personality and because of that she never really happened.*
>
> —Anne Wilson Schaef

We, all too often, are "if" people. We use our "iffing" to try to control our past, our present, and our future.

If only we had been more assertive, we would have made the promotion. *If only* we had been more intelligent, we would have done a better job.

Our "as iffing" tries to cope with the present. We act *as if* we know what we are doing. We act *as if* we are calm and relaxed. After all, we have developed *some* skills!

Yet it is our "what iffing" that really keeps us paralyzed and feeds our illusion that we are in control. We try to imagine every possible exigency and prepare for it before it happens. If I just cover every base, I will never be caught wanting. My "iffing" has resulted in my never being present to my life.

WHEN I QUIT **"iffing,"** I may just start living.

❧ January 21

FEAR

The liar in her terror wants to fill up the void with anything. Her lies are a denial of her fear: a way of maintaining control.

—Adrienne Rich

Our fear is like the first tile in a string of dominoes. Our denial of fear causes us to lie, to cheat, and to become people we don't even respect in order to maintain our illusion of control. We lie because we are fearful, and we are fearful because we lie. It is a circular process and we feel stuck in the middle of these raging feelings.

What a relief it is to admit our fears! What a relief it is to admit that we are powerless over our fears and they are taking over our lives. This admission opens the door to an awareness that if we return to our inner process, our power greater than ourselves, we can feel sane again.

ALL OF US are afraid sometimes, that's human. When our life is ruled by fear, that's obsession.

❧ January 22

OBSTACLES

> *In the upper echelons of the corporate world, it helps to be good-looking . . . but only if you're a man. If you're a woman, attractiveness can be a handicap.*
>
> —Diane Crenshaw

Sometimes it's difficult to accept that the obstacles in our life are there for a purpose and that we have something to learn from them. Some of the obstacles seem so unfair . . . and they are! There still are many double standards operative in the world of business (and elsewhere!) What works for men often doesn't work for women in the same situation. And it isn't fair . . . true . . . and we resent it . . . right . . . as well we should. And while we are trying to change the situation, it is important to see what we have to learn from these unfair obstacles and move on. We don't like them, and it is up to us what we do with them.

OBSTACLES often are not personal attacks; they are muscle builders.

HONESTY

> *When a woman tells the truth she is creating the possibility for more truth around her.*
>
> —Adrienne Rich

Honesty is contagious, just like dishonesty is contagious. We need more honesty in the world.

Many of us have prided ourselves in being honest. We have always tried to be honest and have believed that we were. It has been frightening when we have been told that we are "too honest," or when we have been told that we will not be able to get ahead if we insist on being so "brutally honest." Slowly we have learned to "compromise." We have learned to say what is expected of us and not to offend. We have lost touch with the awareness that we are being dishonest when we go ahead and agree to do something that we really do not feel right about doing. We have come not to expect honesty from ourselves or from those around us. We are even surprised when we encounter it.

IF WE WANT **to heal, we have to start getting honest with ourselves and others. Creating the possibility for more truth is up to each of us.**

INTIMACY

> *. . . just a tender sense of my own inner process, that holds something of my connection with the divine.*
>
> —Shelley

Intimacy, like charity, begins at home. If we cannot be intimate with ourselves, we have no one to bring to intimacy with another person.

Intimacy with ourselves takes time. We need time for rest, time for walks, time for quiet, and time to tune in to ourselves. We cannot completely fill up our lives with activities and become intimate with ourselves. Nor can we just sit quietly indefinitely and become intimate with ourselves. We have to have the time and energy to *be* our lives and to *do* our lives in order to establish an intimate relationship with ourselves.

Surprisingly, as we become intimate with ourselves, we discover our connection with others and with the divine. Neither is possible without intimacy with ourselves.

INTIMACY . . . in/to/me/see. It won't hurt to try it.

LOSING PERSPECTIVE

> *When I am all hassled about something, I always stop and ask myself what difference it will make in the evolution of the human species in the next ten million years, and that question always helps me to get back my perspective.*
> —Anne Wilson Schaef

"Little things mean a lot," especially when we focus all our attention on them, obsess and ruminate about them, and can't let them go. Sometimes we just keep turning disturbing thoughts over and over in our minds, believing that we will surely figure out some solutions if we just think about them long enough and check out every possible angle.

When we engage in this behavior, it is a sure sign that we are thinking ourselves to death. When I do this obsessing, I have lost perspective. I suddenly become the center of the universe, and *my* problems are the only ones that exist.

It always helps me to step back and realize that whatever problem I am having is probably not of universal proportions. This perspective helps me to see that I am powerless over my crazy thinking, and that it is making my life insane. At this point I can get back in touch with my knowing that a power greater than myself can restore me to sanity, and I can turn this problem over to this greater power.

ONE OF THE THINGS we lose when we do too much is perspective.

ANIMALS

> *We're arrogant if we believe we're the only animals with*
> *thoughtful intelligence and an ability to solve problems.*
> *Intelligence also includes feelings, doesn't it? I mean*
> *empathy for others and sadness, also a sense of humor.*
>
> —Jane Goodall

No one who has ever had the privilege of relating to an animal for a period of time can disagree with Jane Goodall. I can't say "anyone who has ever 'owned' an animal," because in relating to an animal it is never quite clear who owns who, and one must question if, indeed, "ownership" comes into the equation at all.

Perhaps it can suffice to say that anyone who has never been in a long-term relationship with an animal has endured and suffered great poverty of the spirit. Nothing is more healing than a warm cat on our laps or a big dog greeting us as we come through the door.

Animals do require time and energy, and all of it is well spent. Animals can be, and usually are, some of our most brilliant and patient teachers. If we want to learn love, devotion, trust, loyalty, responsibility, and many other characteristics we attribute to humans, we can just humbly ask an animal to be our friend.

ONE WHO HAS been chosen for friendship by an animal is a lucky person indeed.

❧ January 27

FORGIVENESS OF MISTAKES

It is very easy to forgive others their mistakes. It takes more gut and gumption to forgive them for having witnessed your own.

—Jessamyn West

How we hate to be seen as our most naked selves! We feel noble when we forgive others their awful mistakes, yet we become paralyzed with guilt and shame when we realize that they have caught us in our worst moments. It is so tempting to try to find something wrong with them and take the focus off what we have done. The best defense is a good offense, we have been told. How hard it is to let ourselves claim and own our mistakes! Yet, also how freeing.

We have the possibility of not only forgiving those who have witnessed our mistakes but also to embrace them as a gift to help keep us honest.

SOMETIMES my gifts are so well-wrapped I have difficulty recognizing them as such. As I unwrap myself, I can unwrap each present.

❧ January 28

EXPENDABLE/CONTROL/FEAR

> *When I was sixteen, my mother told me that I was expendable and if I didn't work hard, companies could just get rid of me. I work sixty to seventy hours a week, never take time off, and my husband and I haven't had a vacation in twelve years. I'm a workaholic, and I love it.*
>
> —Anonymous woman

Whew! Need I say more? This woman has bought the whole package.

Like her, many of us believe that we can control what we perceive as our expendability by making ourselves indispensable. What a sophisticated illusion of control! Obsessive working is different from a passion for our work.

Usually people who are truly passionate about their work are also passionate about their play and their time for themselves. Workaholics are not. We work out of fear and try to convince ourselves that we love it. Fear and self-abuse go together.

AM I **expendable** to *me?* That's the question.

❧ January 29

POWERLESSNESS

> *In the face of an obstacle which is impossible to overcome, stubbornness is stupid.*
>
> —Simone de Beauvoir

Some of us do not like to hear this, but there are some things in our lives over which we are powerless. In fact, when it comes right down to it, there are few aspects of our lives that we can really *control!*

Certainly the areas of our lives over which we are truly the most powerless are our compulsive working, rushing, and busyness habits. We hate the thought of being powerless. As women, we never want to admit to powerlessness again. And maybe *powerlessness is* the right word related to our doing too much. Our inability to stop killing ourselves with doing too much certainly fits into the category of powerlessness whether we like to admit it or not. Paradoxically, admission of powerlessness may restore our personal power.

KNOWING **when to quit may be my greatest victory.**

❧ January 30

MULTI-TASK

It's the multi-tasking that women have to do—from a woman's world. You know, we have to multi-task. I mean 'cause, you know, my getting to work. I get up at 5 o'clock and my trip is a bus route—drop one kid off, drop the next kid off, okay, do I need breakfast? Okay, I'm at work, it's 8 o'clock. I'm not just getting me to work.

—Lucinda

Whew! And she's not a single parent!! Even just listening to the way this young businesswoman shared her "bus route experience" had me exhausted.

She loves her children. She's proud of her children. Yet she is so stressed by the time she gets to work (she has a "no down time" job) that I could only sit there and feel my heart going out to her.

What are we asking of our young women? What are we asking of ourselves? Their mothers and grandmothers worked hard, too, and they had more help than this woman does.

"Doing it all" may mean doing too little for ourselves, our children, our husbands, and our lives.

MAYBE the clue here is in the words "that women *have* to do." When we remember we have choices, we need to make a serious attempt to see that our values inform those choices.

❧ January 31

GIVING OURSELVES AWAY

Somebody almost walked off wid alla my stuff.
                                    —Ntozake Shange

As women, we are often so generous, especially with ourselves, that we give little pieces of ourselves away, to almost anyone who asks. At the time, we hardly notice. Sometimes the pieces we give away are so minuscule that they really seem unimportant . . . a favor here . . . letting something go by that we know is wrong there . . . swallowing the anger from an injustice done to us somewhere else. We can handle each one individually, and we are unaware of the cumulative effect of years of giving away little bits and pieces of ourselves.

We sit up and scream, "*Somebody almost walked off wid alla my stuff!!!*" We have allowed ourselves to be almost devoured by those around us.

GIVING MYSELF AWAY and being stingy are not my only options. I can share myself and not give myself away.

.

❧ February 1

Work as a Sacred Possibility

How is my own life-work serving to end these tyrannies, the corrosions of sacred possibility?

—June Jordan

Sometimes, when we stop to reflect, we need to believe that the work we are doing has a meaning beyond the tedium of the everyday. In fact, if we cannot see some larger connection in what we are doing, we often experience a feeling of loss or emptiness.

We know, somewhere deep inside us, that even if *what* we are doing doesn't exactly have a great cosmic meaning, the *way* we go about it and the interactions we have with others around our work can give it meaning beyond itself. Regardless of what we do, we do have an opportunity to make it sacred work.

I ALWAYS have the freedom for a sacred possibility.

✤ February 2

HAPPINESS

It is not easy to find happiness in ourselves, and it is not possible to find it elsewhere.

—Agnes Repplier

We are the wellspring of our own happiness. Our happiness resides within us. No one else and nothing else can give it to us. We may try to find all kinds of things outside ourselves to fill us up and make us happy, but they are all short-lived. We think success, recognition, respect, money, and prestige will do it for us. They're nice for a while, *and* the feeling lingers that something is missing. This does not mean that a happy person cannot have all these accoutrements of success—she can. Happiness, however, is not a *result* of these symbols of success.

Happiness is ethereal. It only dwells within, and when we seek it, it becomes even more elusive.

I HAVE the opportunity to open myself to the happiness that is mine today and not try to fill myself with happiness substitutes.

❧ February 3

ALONE TIME

And when is there time to remember, to sift, to weigh, to estimate, to total?

—Tillie Olsen

Such a little thing: finding time alone. We have often felt that if we took time for ourselves, we were taking it away from our children, our spouses, or our work and therefore it must be a perversion.

So many little moments during the day are so precious to us. Those few moments after we have sent everyone else off for the day and we can breathe . . . those times alone in the car or on the bus or subway when no one around knows us or can intrude . . . those sighing times in the bathroom when nobody is there . . . even those stolen moments alone while doing the dishes are precious to us.

IT'S ALL RIGHT. **Moments alone and our need for them are not a perversion, they are a life-giving force.**

❧ February 4

GIFTS

Problems are messages.

—Shakti Gawain

I always believe that the intensity of the whack alongside the head that life has to give us in order to get a lesson through to us is directly proportionate to the height and breadth of our stubbornness and illusion of control.

Problems give us the opportunity to learn something. If we don't get the learning the first time around, we get another chance, and another, and another. If we miss the learning completely the first time, the next whack will be a little harder, and then the next time even harder. We get many opportunities to learn the lessons we need to learn in this life.

Obstacles are gifts for learning. We never really know what we have learned until we have learned it. Then we are ready for the next learning.

I HAVE THE OPPORTUNITY **for many gifts today. I hope I see them.**

❧ February 5

EXHAUSTION

Whatever women do they must do twice as well as men to be thought half as good. Luckily, this is not difficult.

—Charlotte Whitton

Although some of us hate to admit it, it is probably true that we have to do things "twice as well as men to be thought half as good." And it is probably also true that we can produce at a level that boggles the mind.

What we tend to ignore is the cost. Working as hard as we do and as long as we do is exhausting. Sometimes we dread becoming aware of how tired we are. Sometimes it almost seems as if the marrow in our bones aches.

Women have a tremendous fear of feeling our tiredness. We are afraid that if we let ourselves feel it, we will never get up again.

MY TIREDNESS is mine. I have earned it.

❧ February 6

BELIEF

Neither reproaches nor encouragements are able to revive a faith that is waning.

—Nathalie Sarraute

Faith, in the last analysis, is a personal process. One of the problems that we as women face in accessing our spiritual self is all the things we have been told that we *should* believe. We have tried to swallow beliefs from outside. Rarely have we taken the time and effort to go inside and start with our own awareness and understanding of God or a power greater than ourselves and let ourselves trust our own knowing. In our busy lives, it is easier to reject than "wait with" our knowing. It is easier to move on than it is to "be with."

No one else can give us the answers about our spirituality. Reading and thinking cannot provide the solutions. Our spirituality is experiential, and it is intimately connected with who we are.

SOMETIMES beliefs have interfered with my connection with a power greater than myself. It is time to "wait with" my knowing.

❧ February 7

The thing that is really hard and really amazing is giving up on being perfect and beginning the work of becoming yourself.

—Anna Quindlen

Perfectionism is an axis around which women who do too much like to spin as we career around our lives. Let's face it, we have had major help and support in our development of our illusion of perfectionism. We have been so indoctrinated in this illusion that we carry it into every aspect of our adult lives.

All too often this illusion of perfectionism—and a difficult and painful illusion it is indeed—feeds another myth, the myth that if we do more we get more done. Together, this illusion of possible perfection and the myth that working longer and harder will produce more result in low production and sloppy work. What a blow!

We always believed that if we did more and more, we would get more done. Wrong. In fact, the opposite is true. The more we push ourselves, the less we get done. *And* the quality of our work suffers.

IT'S DIFFICULT **when illusions and myths crumble (especially when everything around us supports them!), and their crumbling can open the door to new possibilities.**

❧ February 8

MEDICATIONS

I don't have time for pain.

—Tylenol ad

Got a pain? No matter. Take a pill. No time to be sick? Doesn't matter. We have something that will keep you going—and we buy it by the millions. We women who do too much just don't have time for pain.

Pain slows us down. Pain lets us know that something is wrong. Pain interferes with our busy lives. If we can't ignore it, we can medicate it. No problem. Carry on as usual.

Having to take a look at our diet, our destructive "little pleasures," our pushing ourselves too hard would be much too time-consuming and interfere with the things we *have* to get done.

There's one thing we can depend upon. When we create a problem for ourselves, a drug company will step in to develop something to take care of the symptom.

We could, however, take another approach. When we feel pain, we could stop to ask what our bodies are trying to tell us and how we can respond to the pain in a way that will be healing.

WHEN MY BODY gives me warning signals, there are many avenues of responses available to me.

❧ February 9

SUCCESS/GRATITUDE/CLIMBING THE LADDER

Though a tree grow ever so high, the falling leaves return to the ground.

—Malay proverb

Many of us work for and aspire to professional success. We have worked hard and long to get where we are, and we deserve the rewards of our position.

It is important that we periodically take time to take stock of *where* we are and *who* we are. Do we judge ourselves by our accomplishments? Does accomplishment mean worthiness in our book? How have we been able to get where we are, and do we feel good about the way we did it? Do we need to make amends to some people and express our gratitude to others?

It is important to recognize that our achievements not only speak well for us, they speak well for those persons and forces, seen, unseen, and unnoticed, that have been active in our lives.

SUCCESS **offers me the opportunity to reflect on those who have given me much and to be grateful for their gifts.**

❧ February 10

COMMUNICATION

Some people talk simply because they think sound is more manageable than silence.

—Margaret Halsey

Women who do too much need to keep busy. One of the ways we keep busy is talking even when we have nothing to say. It's not that we are so taken with the sound of our own voices. It is just that silence seems so overwhelming and murky.

Much of our lives has been spent filling up . . . overeating and filling up ourselves . . . overworking and filling up our time . . . overtalking and filling up our shared moments of silence.

We need time to be with ourselves in silence.

WHEN PEOPLE TALK on and on, they usually are not listening to themselves.

❧ February 11

ACCEPTANCE/CONFLICT/FEELINGS

When Peter left me, the negative emotions that rose up in me and exploded in me were just horrifying. But God kept telling me that they were all part of me and I couldn't try to hide them under the carpet because I didn't like them.

—Eileen Caddy

There are events in the passage of our lives that elicit feelings we never knew were there and of which we believed *we* were completely incapable. A spouse wants a divorce or has an affair. A boss passes us over for someone younger, prettier (we believe), and less qualified (we know for certain), and we find that the witches of Endor or the dragons of old have nothing on us. We could belch fire and melt diamonds with our breath.

Right, good, so what? It is normal to have feelings like this. It is not healthy to dump them on others or to hold on to them. They will rot inside us.

WHEN I FEEL these feelings, I have another opportunity to learn something new about myself. Thank you ... I think.

February 12

GOALS/COMPETITION

What you have become is the price you paid to get what you used to want.

—Mignon McLaughlin

Was it worth it? Is it worth it? Can we look in the mirror and say to the person we see, "You are someone I trust and really admire"?

We must remember that each step along the road of life is like taking a walk. It gets you somewhere, and steps often leave footprints.

We cannot say to ourselves, "Well, what I am doing is expedient now, so I will go ahead and do it this way. I will deal with the consequences later," and not *have* consequences later. The denials of our life are interrelated.

WHAT I DO becomes who I am. I am working with precious elements here.

❧ February 13

PERSONAL MORALITY

I cannot and will not cut my conscience to fit this year's fashions.

—Lillian Hellman

One of the effects of doing too much is that we gradually lose contact with our personal morality and we slowly deteriorate as a moral person. It is easy to see how the alcoholic or drug addict is progressively willing to lie, cheat, steal, and even kill or hurt the one she loves in order to get her fix. But women who do too much are not so different. We have moral slippage too. We will withhold information, lie, mislead, or undercut others to get ahead. We are willing to compromise our standards and our morality to get to the top, to "fit this year's fashions." When we compromise our personal morality, we have sold our souls and we are losing the "us which is us."

We need to recognize that our personal morality is one of our most precious assets and too important to treat lightly.

I VALUE myself enough to realize that my personal morality is a beacon that demands to be followed.

❧ February 14

EXPECTATIONS

> *Nobody objects to a woman being a good writer or sculptor or geneticist if at the same time she manages to be a good wife, good mother, good-looking, good-tempered, well-groomed and unaggressive.*
>
> —Leslie M. McIntyre

Right! So what's the problem? It's not easy to be well-groomed when we have toddlers running around . . . but we try. It's not easy to be good-tempered and unaggressive when we have deadlines at work and at home . . . but we try. It is not easy to produce children and be svelte and good-looking . . . but we try.

There is probably no group of people in this society who try harder than women to meet the expectations of others. As a result, we are always looking outside for validation, and no matter how much we get, it isn't enough. In always trying to be what others think we should be, we have lost ourselves and end up having little to bring to any relationship or task.

EXPECTATIONS are like girdles. We probably should have discarded them years ago.

FEELING CRAZY

> *You can't start worrying about what's going to happen. You*
> *get spastic enough worrying about what's happening now.*
> —Lauren Bacall

Why is it that *we* always seem to be the ones that need the help. We do feel crazy at times, and feelings of being overwhelmed are not unfamiliar. And yet, why does the label craziness (if someone has to be crazy!) always rest on us?

Sometimes, it's a relief to admit that we feel crazy. Sometimes, we do need someone to talk with when we feel isolated. Others appear to cope all right. Why can't we? At least, talking with someone or going to a group with other women helps us recognize that we are not alone in these feelings. Seeking out help and support can be a real turning point.

PERHAPS my inability to cope with an insane situation the way I always used to be able to is a sign of my movement toward health.

❧ February 16

TIME

We need to exercise. We're supposed to look good all the time. I try to do it two-three times a week, but still, just walking an hour is about all you can get, and that's hard.

So, really, getting up earlier in the morning before you start your day—or at the end of the day when everybody's asleep. Then—then all you want to do is sleep. That's about it. There's no time.

—Mary

There's no time. There's no time. There's no time. This seems to be a modern mantra. I have an elder friend in Ireland who once said to me, "God made time—and he made plenty of it." That old adage stopped me in my tracks.

Hmmm. It's not that we don't *have* enough time. There's plenty of it.

There's plenty of it. Now there's a concept to be reckoned with. God made all the time we need. We *have* all the time we need. Can I dare believe that reality?

IT'S NOT that God didn't give us all the time we need. It's what *we* have *done* with time that is giving us a problem.

❧ February 17

AWARENESS OF
PROCESS/CONTROL/CREATIVITY

Living in process is being open to insight and encounter. Creativity is becoming intensively absorbed in the process and giving it form.

—Susan Smith

When we choose to live our lives in a process way, we choose to be open to all that life has to offer. Our illusion of control has often filtered out new insights and encounters. We have been so focused upon our goals and the way things *have* to happen, that we have missed the succulent serendipity of chance awarenesses. We have been so afraid of losing our illusion of control that we have missed some of the richest encounters that life was offering us.

When we can participate fully in the process of our lives, we discover new forms of our creative self. Creativity has many avenues. Just living our lives can cultivate our conscious creativity.

CAN IT BE? Is just living my life enough?

❧ February 18

FRANTIC

> *We have come to a place where frantic and panic seem integral to being a woman, especially a professional woman.*
>
> —Anne Wilson Schaef

Women who do too much tend to get frantic over almost anything. Where *did* we park that rental car at the airport and what in the world did it look like anyway? We were *sure* that we parked our own car right in front of the drugstore at the shopping mall. Or was that last week?

Where did we put that bill that simply must be paid today? There must be a way to get the kids off in the morning that could be less frantic. We are *sure* an organized mother could do better.

Where is that pen? Where is that pan? Where are those pants? Probably right where we left them. It is usually our "frantic" that clouds our vision.

FRANTIC AND PANIC **are old familiar friends. Maybe it is time for them to move out of our house.**

JUGGLING PROJECTS

We are traditionally rather proud of ourselves for having slipped creative work in there between the domestic chores and obligations. I'm not sure we deserve such big A-pluses for all that.

—Toni Morrison

Women who work outside the house aren't the only women who are obsessed with work. Women who are home full-time rarely have time for themselves and their creative projects either. After all, children are twenty-four hours a day and the house is twenty-four hours a day. There is always something to do.

Our greatest skill is not perhaps in getting things done, it may be in juggling projects so it looks like we are getting things done, so that we feel better. Watch out! Juggling projects is one of the symptoms of those who do too much. Instead of paring down the projects to those that can reasonably be done, we try to do it all.

JUGGLERS aren't paid very well, and sometimes they get hit on the head with balls they have in the air.

❧ February 20

AMENDS

> *Make it a rule of life never to regret and never look back.*
> *Regret is an appalling waste of energy; you can't build on*
> *it; it is good only for wallowing in.*
>
> —Katherine Mansfield

Looking back and regretting are very different from taking stock, making amends, and moving on. When we look back and regret, we are indulging in the self-centered activity of beating up on ourselves over the mistakes in our past.

All of us have made mistakes. When we have operated out of the craziness of doing too much, we have done much harm to ourselves and others. We have neglected ourselves. We have neglected those we love. That is the nature of doing too much. Now we can admit our wrongs, make amends to those we have wronged (including amends to ourselves when we have not been caring for ourselves), and move on.

We cannot build on shame, guilt, or regret. We, indeed, can only wallow in them.

OWNING **and making amends for my mistakes affords me the opportunity to build on my past and integrate it. I can start doing this anytime . . . maybe even today.**

VALUES

> *When women take on a career, they don't discard their female values, but add them onto the traditional male values of work achievement and career success. As they struggle to fill the demands of both roles, women can't understand why men don't share this dual value system.*
> —Susan Sturdinent and Gail Donoff

One of the often most painful learnings for women who work outside the home is that the same skills that work in business just do not work in our homes and in our personal relationships. Luckily, we have the advantage of knowing a value system that does contribute to living, and we have only to learn what works at work.

Unfortunately, in the process of learning a career value system, we are encouraged to denigrate our values and sometimes we succumb to this pressure. Our values are not wrong. They are different. And the workplace would be richer with them.

TRUSTING **my value system can be a major contribution to my work.**

❧ February 22

SOLITUDE

Thrice welcome, friendly Solitude,
let no busy foot intrude,
Nor listening ear be nigh!
　　　　—Hester Chapone, from *Ode to Solitude*

Solitude is such a blessing! Everyone needs time alone. Often we are fearful of time alone, because there is no one for us to encounter but ourselves. How comforting it is to go to ourselves! How much like returning home to an old friend or lover after having been away too long visiting places that felt foreign and unfamiliar.

Our solitude is one of the pleasures that only we can arrange. It is up to us to see that we regenerate through our time with ourselves. We have the right, and we have the power. If we do not model respect for our own need for solitude, our children will never learn that they deserve their time alone.

LET ME REMEMBER that I have the right to create a space of solitude for myself, if only to enjoy the soothing sound of running water in my own bathtub.

❧ February 23

LETTING GO

> *Foggy thinking, dizziness, and recurring headaches may be signals that it is time to let go of something in your life that isn't working.*

—Christiane Northrup

Isn't working! Isn't working, you say? When something isn't working, let it go. What a preposterous idea!

We women who do too much often see something that isn't working as a call to arms. We can work a little harder. Push a little harder. Do a bit more. TRY HARDER, TRY harder, try harder. . . . Isn't letting go the same as giving up?

Life in its normal state is a series of cycles, a series of beginnings and endings, a series of changes. We humans are probably the only species willing to make ourselves sick by holding on to something that has already passed.

It's very strange that often, when we are *willing* to let go, truly willing, then everything shifts and letting go may not be the issue. Our holding on may make us sick.

LETTING GO **is usually a statement of personal power, not a defeat.**

CHOICES/RESPONSIBILITY

We're swallowed up only when we are willing for it to happen.

—Nathalie Sarraute

When we talk about taking responsibility for our lives, we must clarify what we mean by responsibility. The cultural meaning of the word *responsibility* means accountability and blame. When women accept that meaning, they cannot bear to take responsibility for their lives or to see other women do so, because, they assume, taking responsibility means taking the *blame* for where they are and who they are. Unfortunately, this attitude puts us in the position of being victims and robbing us of our power.

It is only when we accept that we do have choices, and we exercise those choices, that we can reclaim our lives. Inherent in this reclaiming process is owning the choices we have made (all of them!) and moving on. Thus we are not blaming ourselves for our lives; we are claiming them and owning them so we can take our next steps.

I HAVE MADE some bad choices, I have made some so-so choices, and I have made some good choices. The most important aspect of them is that they are mine—all of them.

❧ February 25

PAIN

> *Iron, left in the rain*
> *And fog and dew,*
> *With rust is covered.—Pain*
> *Rusts into beauty too.*

> —Mary Carolyn Davies

Our pain is ours. Some of it we have earned, the rest not, and it is still ours. When we fight our pain, we fight the experience of our humanness, and we lose ourselves in the process. A life without pain is a life of nonliving. Our pain lets us know and come to understand the full meaning of being human. If we fight the normal experience of our pain, we lose the possibility to experience the process of its rusting "into beauty too."

We don't need to seek pain, but when it is inevitably there, we have the possibility of something new entering our lives.

MY PAIN is a possibility. It is not a liability or a punishment.

❧ February 26

NURTURING ONESELF

Just the knowledge that a good book is awaiting one at the end of a long day makes that day happier.

—Kathleen Norris

The art of nurturing oneself is not something that is taught in most high schools or even in a good MBA (Master of Business Administration) course. In fact, the art of nurturing oneself is rarely taught in families either.

Yet, in this high-tech, high-information society, learning how to nurture oneself is absolutely essential for survival. Some of us have found that if we do a cursory job of nurturing ourselves, we can work even harder. Unfortunately, that isn't nurturing oneself, that's protecting one's supply.

Nurturing oneself is allowing ourselves to stop, and in that stopping to allow ourselves to know what would be nurturing for us in that time and space, and doing it.

WHAT IS NURTURING at one point in our lives may not be nurturing at another. In order to nurture myself, I have to know myself each moment.

✽ February 27

PERFECTIONISM

> *This is the age of perfectionism, kid.*
> *Everybody try their emotional and mental and*
> *physical damndest.*
> Strive, strive. Correct all defects.

> —Judith Guest

Perfectionism is one of the characteristics of doing too much. Perfectionism is setting up an abstract, external ideal of what we should be or should be able to do that has little or no relationship to who we are or what we need to do and then trying to mold ourselves into that ideal.

In trying to be the abstract perfect, we batter, judge, and distort ourselves. No matter what we do or how we try to achieve, it is never enough. We are never enough. Trying too hard and never trying at all are two sides of the coin of perfection. Unfortunately, it is a coin that never pays off.

PERFECTIONISM **is self-abuse of the highest order.**

❧ February 28

LAUGHTER

Laughter can be more satisfying than honor; more precious than money; more heart-cleansing than prayer.

—Harriet Rochlin

How long has it been since you have had a good belly laugh? Good laughter seems to be a treasure that is in short supply of late.

Most of us are distrustful and embarrassed by our laughter. As children we were constantly told to suppress it. Often it seems almost lost to us. We are afraid to laugh alone, and we are embarrassed to laugh with others. What a state!

Laughter is one of the gifts of being human. We can't force it, but we can sure stop suppressing it in ourselves and in our children.

LAUGHTER is like the human body wagging its tail.

❧ February 29

IMPRESSION MANAGEMENT

> *And yet, all these years I'd been terrified I would be stoned to death if people saw through the facade.*
>
> —Sara Davidson

How much time and energy we spend in impression management! We firmly believe that if we just dress right others (especially men) will think we are professional, intelligent, competent, and in control. We believe that if we just dress right others (usually men) will think we are attractive, sexy, desirable, and worth knowing. We think that if we are just caring, understanding, and constant enough someone will want to be with us.

We have such terror that someone will see through our facade and discover (our greatest fear!) that no one is there. We believe that if people really know who we are, they would have no interest in us. We believe that it is our impression management that keeps us safe.

OF COURSE, if someone falls in love with my impression, they aren't loving me, they're only loving my image.

❧ March 1

IN TOUCH WITH PROCESS/GREATER POWER

We both of us secretly believed in an external power that one could tap, if one were in tune with events.

—Robyn Davidson

Living in process is living *our* process and being one with the process of the universe. Our busyness removes us from our connection with the living process. Our busyness alienates us from our spirituality and our faith and tells us we aren't safe, we have to control, and we must try to assure security by making ourselves, our lives, and even the universe static.

We put so much effort into trying to make our universe static that we have not developed the capacity to be in tune with events. As we learn to tune in and participate, we find that living our process is so much easier than trying to make the universe static.

WHEN I am in touch with my process, I am in touch with the process of the universe.

❧ March 2

FEELING CRAZY

Feeling crazy may be a mark of sanity in my situation.
—Anne Wilson Schaef

Several years ago, after I had written and published *Women's Reality,* I visited an old friend in New York City. After talking a while, she said, "You've changed." (She's an analyst and she always notices things!) "Really," I said, "How?" (I secretly hoped that I had changed. After all, we had not seen each other for several years, and if I hadn't changed, I was in deep trouble!) "You are no longer afraid of being crazy," she observed. "Was I afraid I was crazy?" I asked, somewhat startled. "Yes," she said quietly. "Well, after writing *Women's Reality,* I realize that I have constantly been told that I am crazy by my society when I put forth my clearest, sanest, most precious perceptions. Now I accept that I am 'crazy' in the eyes of an insane society, and I feel very 'sane' with my 'craziness.'"

WATCH OUT for who is defining "crazy."

✸ March 3

LETTING GO/RESENTMENTS

Wanna fly, you got to give up the shit that weighs you down.

—Toni Morrison

Our old "shit" is so precious to us. We tenderly harbor our old resentments and periodically throw them pieces of fresh flesh to keep them alive. We nurture our anger. We don't do anything to work it through or let it go, we just hang on and nurture it. And we wonder why we feel so stuck and held back in our lives.

When we hold on to old resentment, it weighs us down. It is as if our feet are stuck in fresh tar.

There comes a time when we can see that it doesn't really matter what someone has done to us, our holding on to it is hurting us, not them, and if we want to heal, we had best take our old anger and fertilize the flowers.

THE ONLY WAY **to grow is to let go.**

❧ March 4

FEELINGS/FREEDOM

The white fathers told us, "I think therefore I am," and the Black mother within each of us—the poet—whispers in our dreams, I feel, therefore I can be free.

—Audre Lorde

We have been trained to shut off and freeze our feelings. We have been told that feelings are weak and irrational and if we want to be a success in this world, we must be able to control our feelings. The models for success are persons who never have any visible feelings.

Yet when we do this, we find that we are making ourselves more vulnerable, not less. When we push feelings down, we never know when or how they will erupt, and we can rest assured that it will be with greater intensity than if we had acknowledged the original "feeling moment."

Also, feelings are our natural, built-in alarm and information system. It is our feelings not our minds that warn us of danger, that tell us that someone is lying to us, and that tell us of subtle nuances that allow us to discern differences and make decisions. Without this internal information system we can never truly be free.

CELEBRATING **my ability to feel is a way to be fully free.**

❧ March 5

LONELINESS

Loneliness and the feeling of being unwanted is the most terrible poverty.

—Mother Teresa

The feeling of loneliness is not uncommon to women who do too much. We are constantly busy and surrounded by people and still we feel lonely. In fact, it is quite possible that one of the reasons that we keep so busy is that we are trying to avoid our feelings of loneliness and are, simultaneously, frightened by intimacy.

We believe if we just rush around enough, keep busy enough, and surround ourselves with enough important and interesting people, our loneliness will disappear. Unfortunately, none of these things works. Indeed, as Fiona Macleod says, "My heart is a lonely hunter that hunts on a lonely hill." Our hearts are seeking something, and the many things we have tried don't seem to be it. When we have lost the connection with our spiritual beings, we will be lonely no matter how much we have.

LONELINESS **is not outside, it's inside.**

❧ March 6

It has been wisely said that we cannot really love any-
body at whom we never laugh.

—Agnes Repplier

How serious we are about everything—especially relationships! Often in our most intimate possibilities, we forget that our laughter at ourselves and at each other is one of the vehicles that our creator has given us for grounding ourselves in reality. And relationships that are not grounded in reality don't last.

We have to know others very well to be able to see their funny sides and to share in the frivolity of family functions. Let's face it, we human beings are a funny lot. No robot has ever been capable of the antics we can think up.

SHARING **my laughter at myself and others is one of the ways threads of intimacy are spun.**

❧ March 7

SANITY

> *If, as someone has said, ". . . to be truly civilized, is to embrace disease . . ."*

—Robyn Davidson

One of the by-products of living and working in crazy situations is that our tolerance for insanity increases exponentially. Our ability to discern what makes sense and what doesn't becomes impaired. When those around us continually exhibit bizarre behavior, we begin to question our sanity. Often we are not insane. The situation is insane, and we become progressively crazy as we try to adjust to it.

If "to be truly civilized, is to embrace disease," maybe we need to take a look at what we have defined as "civilized."

I AM NOT CRAZY—it's just that my situation seems to require a crazy person.

SELF-AFFIRMATION

> *i found God in myself*
> *& i loved her/i loved her fiercely.*

> —Ntozake Shange

What better place to find God than within ourselves! It is only when we really know ourselves and affirm ourselves for who we are that we become aware of the divinity that we share with all things. We are part of the hologram . . . we *are* the hologram. When we estrange ourselves from ourselves, we also then lose contact with that which is beyond ourselves.

To know "God" and to love her fiercely is to love ourselves. Loving this God is not loving the self-centered "God" of confusion. It is loving the God that is one, that is within us, and beyond us. It is loving God as we understand God.

CONTACT **with God is so simple, and we make it so difficult.**

❧ March 9

SELF-ESTEEM/HIGHER POWER

Part of my satisfaction and exultation at each eruption was unmistakably feminist solidarity. You men think you're the only ones that can make a really nasty mess? You think you got all the firepower and God's on your side? You think you run things? Watch this, gents. Watch the Lady act like a woman.

—Ursula K. Le Guin

In some surprising way, Mount Saint Helens proved to be an important symbol for all of us. She reminded us of powers that are unseen and uncontrolled. She reminded us that there are forces on this planet and in this universe over which we have no control. We not only had no control over her eruptions, we could not even predict what she was going to do next, even though we applied our best scientific technology and kept her under constant surveillance. She demonstrated to our technocratic society that nature (often identified as female, especially when she's "bad") could not be controlled.

Although none of us wants destruction to occur or lives to be lost, we do need occasionally to be reminded that we are not in charge.

WHEN SHE SIMMERS silently, she is like a woman. When she blows her top off, she is like a woman. We have a range of responses.

SERENITY

> *I am suddenly filled with that sense of peace and meaning which is, I suppose, what the pious have in mind when they talk about the practice of the presence of God.*
>
> —Valerie Taylor

The word *serenity* is something that we understand in abstract and often not in practice. As we begin to take care of ourselves and recover from our compulsive doing, we begin to experience *moments* of serenity. The first time we experience serenity, it may zip through our consciousness like a meteor and scare us to death, because this feeling of serenity is so foreign to us. After a while, we begin to recognize these moments of serenity as very special, and we try to *make* them happen through rituals, practices, and techniques. We are now not focusing on controlling the world, we are trying to control our experience of serenity . . . back to the drawing board. Control is control.

SERENITY is a gift. It is available to all of us. It is being one with the presence of God.

❧ March 11

STRAIGHTENING THE HOUSE/REGRET

My tidiness and my untidiness are full of regret and remorse and complex feelings.

—Natalia Ginzburg

One of the greatest gifts that my mother gave me was that she was a *terrible* housekeeper. She wasn't terrible at everything, she just was terrible at keeping the house clean, which she firmly believed that she should be able to do.

She was a published poet, a great writer of short stories, a painter, a talented breaker and trainer of horses, an avid reader, a knowledgeable collector of antiques, a seeker into the psychic and the mysteries of the world, a good mother, a true, loyal, and devoted friend, incurably curious, an authority on American Indian lore, an intuitive searcher for precious rocks, fossils, and old gems, a defender of everyone's civil rights, and most of all a fascinating and extraordinary woman, but she couldn't keep the kitchen floor clean.

I was not at all damaged by the state of our house. I was saddened that she sometimes negatively judged who she was. *And*, she freed me from worrying about my house and how clean it was or wasn't.

IF NOTHING ELSE, I hope I can remember what is important in this life.

❧ March 12

ACCEPTANCE/MISTAKES/AMENDS

*Of all the idiots I have met in my life, and the Lord
knows that they have not been few or little, I think that
I have been the biggest.*

—Isak Dinesen

One of the ways that I can reclaim my power and my
person is to admit my mistakes. Sometimes it is helpful
to sit down and make a list of people that I have
wronged (including myself) and to make amends to
those with whom it is possible and where it would not
harm them to do so.

What a clean feeling it is to accept and own my life
and not beat myself up for the mistakes I have made!
How good it feels to let those I have harmed know that
I am aware of what I have done and that I genuinely
wish to own and change my behavior, and do what I can
to live clearer and cleaner in the future.

ADMITTING our mistakes and making amends are powerful tools for reclaiming ourselves.

❧ March 13

SPIRITUAL LIFE

> *We are not human beings trying to be spiritual. We are spiritual beings trying to be human.*
>
> —Jacquelyn Small

So often we try to compartmentalize our spirituality and therefore (hopefully) keep it under control. Our spirituality is much more all-encompassing than many of us care to admit. Everything we do flows from ourselves as spiritual beings. When we make decisions, our spirituality is there. When we interact at work, our spirituality is there. When we wash the dishes our spirituality is there. So often we have tried to remove our spiritual selves from our daily selves because we equated spirituality with saintliness, and we did not always want saintliness interfering with our daily lives. It is only when we recognize that all that we do is spiritual, that we can let our spirituality inform our humanity.

NOTHING I DO **is too tiny or too tedious to be spiritual.**

❧ March 14

ANGER

Fury gathered until I was swollen with it.

—Vera Randal

How many of us know that fury that rises like a thermometer within us until our vocal cords quiver and our eyes turn a bright red and then glaze over? Young children and animals always know to scatter at times like these.

Some of us roll up the windows and scream in our cars on the highways. Some of us wait until no one is around and scream into our pillows. Some of us just scream. Most of us have thought we were crazy at these times. We're not. We are just alive and responding to our stressful lives.

A GOOD scream-a-logue not directed at anyone is often much more effective than a dialogue.

❧ March 15

ALONE TIME

When we, as individuals, first rediscover our spirit, we are usually drawn to nurture and cultivate this awareness.

—Shakti Gawain

Alone time is absolutely essential to the human organism. Many of us have been afraid to be alone. We are afraid that if someone else is not around, no one will be present. When we have lost the awareness of ourselves, we try to fill up our time with work, busyness, food, and other people. We have been afraid to sound our own depths. We have been afraid that we would look inside and find no one there.

Yet, when we have that first awareness of "rediscovering our spirit," we know that there is someone there, inside of us, who is well worth knowing.

There is no way to know ourselves unless we have time alone to explore. We need to nurture and protect our alone time even when it seems difficult.

MY ALONE TIME is as essential to my spirit as food, sleep, and exercise are to my body. I hope I am able to remember that.

TEARS

> *I have been told that crying makes me seem soft and therefore of little consequence. As if our softness has to be the price we pay out for power, rather than simply the one that's paid most easily and most often.*
>
> —Audre Lorde

Our tears and our softness are not valued much in this society, especially in the workplace. In the past, women have been led to believe that we could gain indirect, manipulative power through our tears and our gentle willingness to take care of others.

Many modern women have rejected using our tears and our gentleness to get what we want. Unfortunately, this rejection of our gentler side has resulted in our trying to appear tough and aggressive and in our losing our wholeness.

We are neither all soft nor all tough. We just are.

SHARING my tears and softness is an act of love. Sharing my strength and assertiveness is also an act of love. When I share me, I am loving.

❧ March 17

BECOMING/ACCEPTANCE

The great thing about getting older is that you don't lose all the other ages you've been.

—Madeline L'Engle

Life is a process. We are a process. Everything that has happened in our lives has happened for a reason and is an integral part of our becoming.

One of the challenges of our lives is to integrate the pieces of our lives as we live them. It is sometimes tempting to try to deny huge periods of our lives or forget significant events, especially if they have been painful. To try to erase our past is to rob ourselves of our own hard-earned wisdom.

There is not a child or an adolescent within us. There is the child or adolescent who has grown into us.

When we realize that among the most important strengths that we bring to our work are the life experiences we have had and the ages we have been, maybe we will not resent getting older.

MY WISDOM emerges as I accept and integrate all that I have been and all that has happened to me.

AWARENESS

For me, it's a constant discipline to remember to go back inside to connect with my intuition.

—Shakti Gawain

Each of us has much more brainpower than we ever use. We have so overdeveloped the logical/rational/linear parts of our brains that we frequently have left undeveloped our awareness, intuition, and creativity. We sometimes even forget that awareness, intuition, and creativity *are* brain functions.

Yet, even without being valued and exercised, these aspects of our selves remain faithful and do not leave us. Whenever we open ourselves to our intuition, it is always there. It is important that we remember to go back inside to connect with our intuition. Trusting our intuition often saves us from disaster.

IT IS SOMETIMES **frightening to trust my intuition. It is always disastrous *not* to trust it.**

UNREALISTIC PROMISES/DESPAIR

We workaholics make so many promises that no human being could possibly keep them. That is one of the ways we keep ourselves feeling bad about ourselves.

—Lynn

One of the problems that we workaholics and care-aholics have is that we overextend ourselves and believe that we can and should be able to fulfill the promises we make. We want to be nice. We want to be members of the team. We want to be seen as competent and dependable.

We also hate to say no when someone notices us and has the confidence in us to ask us to do something. We *want* to be able to deliver.

Yet, when we do not check out with ourselves whether we can or want to fulfill our promises, we end up overcommitting ourselves and ultimately feeling bad about ourselves, which just feeds our self-esteem problems.

CHECKING **to see if I can and want to fulfill a promise before I make it is good for me and good for others.**

FEELINGS/CONTROL

> *For years I have endeavored to calm an impetuous tide—laboring to make my feelings take an orderly course—it was striving against the stream.*
>
> —Mary Wollstonecraft

We have generally been taught that feelings are bad. They aren't logical and rational. They are unruly, messy, unpredictable, and often intense. How wonderful to have such a range of expression!

Often, as children, it was not just our feelings of anger, rage, sadness, or pouting that were stifled. We were told to be quiet and equally commanded to suppress our feelings of excitement, joy, creativity, imagination, giggles, laughter, and happiness. Strangely enough, we have found that it is not possible to suppress some feelings and not others. When we push down anger, joy goes with it. When we push down rage, tenderness goes with it.

We are often told as adults that our anger must be appropriate, nonoffensive, justified, and expressed in the right way. What a joke. Trying to girdle my feelings is like trying to tie down the wind.

WHEN I ignore and suppress my feelings, they come out in frightening, sometimes destructive ways. I need to learn to honor them . . . whatever they are.

❧ March 21

FORGIVENESS

If you haven't forgiven yourself something, how can you forgive others?

—Dolores Huerta

Forgiveness has to start with the self. To forgive ourself does not mean that we condone or support everything we have done. It means that we own it. We claim it. We accept that we were in the wrong, and we move on.

Often, when we recognize that we are in the wrong, we slip into our self-centeredness, becoming so absorbed and arrogant in berating ourselves that we never quite reach a stage of forgiveness. To forgive we have to let go and move on. If we do not know how to do that with ourselves, we can never forgive others.

"TO ERR is human, to forgive divine." To forgive myself and others is divinely human.

❧ March 22

PATIENCE/DECISIONS

*Our most important decisions are discovered, not made.
We can make the unimportant ones but the major ones
require us to wait with the discovery.*

— Anne Wilson Schaef

We often push ourselves to decisions that have not ripened and are not ready to be made. We castigate ourselves for being indecisive, and others share this opinion of us. We believe that if we were just wise enough, intelligent enough, or clear enough we would know what we want. We do not respect that maybe the reason we can't make a decision is because we *don't know yet*.

For many generations, women have felt that we had to say yes to everything. Then we learned that it is OK to say no, so we have practiced saying no. Unfortunately, however, it is still exceedingly difficult for us to say "I don't know" and to feel comfortable staying with our not knowing, until we do know.

THE QUALITY of my decisions is directly proportionate to my patience with my not knowing.

HANGING IN THERE

To be somebody you must last.

—Ruth Gordon

We women who do too much know how to "hang in there." We stick with a situation that a sane person would have given up on years ago. This persistence is, indeed, often a part of our insanity. We get so fixated on hanging in that we lose perspective and fail to see that our very persistence may be exacerbating a sick situation. If we withdraw from the situation, organizations in which we are involved might have the opportunity to test their reality, or they may even be allowed to "hit bottom" and come out the other side.

We accept the virtue of perseverance but unfortunately our dedication to it has affected our judgment and our ability to discern what is really needed.

IN SOME situations it is better to leave; in some it is important to persevere, in some we simply have to wait and see. The trick is to discern which is which.

❧ March 24

GRATITUDE

> *You love like a coward. Don't take no steps at all. Just stand around and hope for things to happen outright. Unthankful and unknowing like a hog under an acorn tree. Eating and grunting with your ears hanging over your eyes, and never even looking up to see where the acorns are coming from.*
>
> —Zora Neale Hurston

So often we go through life like hogs. We root around and munch on the goodies around us without ever once acknowledging where they come from or that we are receiving them as gifts.

The process of the universe is so generous with us that we take too much for granted. We "love like cowards." We expect everyone and everything around us to take risks, while we *take*. We become so arrogant that we convince ourselves that everything that we have is a gift from us to us. We don't stop to see that we couldn't be munching those tasty acorns unless there were some celestial oak tree dropping them.

TODAY, **I have the opportunity to stop, look up, and be grateful for the many gifts that are mine.**

❧ March 25

BUSYNESS

> *My husband and I have figured out a really good system about the housework: neither one of us does it.*
>
> —Dottie Archibald

I wonder if this would work. Have I ever had the courage and security to let my housework go for several years, to see if there was a natural limit to the amount of dirt that accumulated? Nope, and I'm not sure I want to.

Yet, how much of the constant repetitive housework I do is because of my need to keep busy and not because it actually needs to be done?

One of the characteristics of a person who does too much is procrastination. Often, our busyness is a subtle form of procrastination that keeps us away from what we *really* need to be doing.

I AM GRATEFUL for the things I hear that give me the opportunity to shift my perception ever so slightly.

❧ March 26

COURAGE/FEAR

Courage—fear that has said its prayers.

—Dorothy Bernard

I wonder if it is possible to be in touch with our true courageousness without being in touch with our spirituality? We know how to be foolhardy. We know how to take risks. We even know how to put ourselves on the line.

But do we know how to soar through the tempering fires of our fear, reach deep into our spirit, and find the courage that is there? Do we have the courage for the dailiness of life? Can we admit a mistake and not give in to the luxury of self-castigation? Do we have the courage to be honest about who we really are with those we love? Do we have the courage to return a bad piece of meat to the butcher, or do we just grumble? Do we have the courage to take a nap?

When we face our fears and let ourselves know our connection to the power that is in us and beyond us, we learn courage.

MY COURAGE is everyday, just like my spirituality. Everyday courage is all I ask.

❧ March 27

DISCOURAGEMENT

> *Only the dusty flowers, the clank of censers and tracks,*
> *leading from somewhere to nowhere.*
>
> —Anna Akhmatova

What a beautiful expression of discouragement! . . . Tracks that lead from somewhere to nowhere. We have all tried so hard to do the right things. We have gone to the right schools, followed the rules, worked long hours, skipped long showers . . . and for what? . . . tracks that lead from somewhere (with dusty flowers along the way) to nowhere, or perhaps even tracks that lead from nowhere to nowhere.

Relax. Of course we feel discouraged at times. Growth is more like a spiral than a line. Our struggles offer us the opportunity to become better acquainted with the many facets of our doing too much.

GROWTH **doesn't have to be a straight line. As long as I am on the road, I must be going somewhere.**

DESPAIR

> *If God is a fly on the wall, Nanny, hand me a flyswatter.*
> —Gaby Brimmer

Even Jesus felt forsaken by God. We can identify with him. We have been angry with God, and we have abandoned our Higher Power because we felt abandoned. This God on whom we want to depend simply refuses to live our lives for us. We want to turn it all over to our Higher Power and lie back and relax, and old H.P. is not cooperating.

Where's the flyswatter? If my Higher Power won't do it my way, to hell with it.

Right! Enjoying ourselves, are we? Isn't this fun? A fight with God—that should keep us occupied for quite some time.

WHEN I FEEL **abandoned by my Higher Power, I am the one who has gone away.**

PASSION

> *It is the soul's duty to be loyal to its own desires. It must
> abandon itself to its master passion.*
>
> —Rebecca West

Many competent women have a difficult time distinguishing between passion and workaholism. When we hear the emerging concern about the lethal effects of compulsive working, we almost always ask ourselves (or justify to ourselves): "But what about being passionate with my work? Are you saying that to be passionate about my work is to be a workaholic? I don't want to give up my work."

Many of our role models for success are people who were willing to be devoured by their work. This is confusing to us.

True passion and doing what is important for us to do does not require us to destroy ourselves in the process. In fact, it is when passion gets distorted to compulsivity that it is destructive.

MY PASSION feeds me. My doing too much devours me. There is a great difference between the two.

❧ March 30

BECOMING

A clay pot sitting in the sun will always be a clay pot. It has to go through the white heat of the furnace to become porcelain.

—Mildred Witte Stouven

Actually, there's nothing wrong with being a clay pot. It's just that all of us have the potential to become porcelain. And it isn't quite so simple as just being fired or not being fired. Some of us explode in the kiln. Some of us collapse before we ever reach the kiln, and some of us develop horrible cracks that seriously threaten our utilitarian value.

Yet probably the saddest response is to have gone through the firing and to refuse to become porcelain. All of us have furnaces in our lives. Not all of us glean the lessons from the firing.

IT IS OUR FAITH that facilitates our surrender to the firing.

MEANNESS/MEAN-SPIRITEDNESS

Such an attractive lass. So outdoorsy. She loves nature in spite of what it did to her.

—Bette Midler

Women who do too much tend to develop an edge that can be cutting at times. Let's face it. When we feel so tired, strung out, and pulled in so many directions we start to get a little ragged around the edges without even knowing it. Even our attempts at humor can become mean-spirited.

When this mean-spiritedness occurs, we aren't funny. We're cruel. And even though people may laugh at our remarks, they also will probably emotionally take a few steps back and put up a bit of a protective shield. Deep down, even if we usually enjoy our own humor, we feel uncomfortable with ourselves when we are mean-spirited.

MEANNESS and mean-spiritedness are good warning signs for us to notice that we are becoming persons we don't like or want to be. We had better take notice.

✣ April 1

GIFTS

April
Comes like an idiot, babbling, and strewing flowers.
                              —Edna St. Vincent Millay

One of the gifts of life is the changing of the weather and the seasons. As we relinquish some of our illusions of control, we realize that each change of the weather and each season of the year have many gifts in store for us, if we participate in them and live with them. When we fight and struggle against the weather and the seasons, we dissipate the energy that could be used for enjoyment.

April does seem to enter "like an idiot" sometimes . . . a playful, energetic, sparkling idiot that brings in riots . . . riots of flowers. Summer gives us longer days to enjoy and a time for laziness, if we accept the offers of summer. Fall gathers in, and winter cozies in. In living with the seasons, we receive many gifts.

ACCEPTING **nature's gift of the seasons is like opening brightly colored packages loosely tied with crinkled ribbons.**

❧ April 2

LIVING LIFE FULLY

Don't be afraid your life will end: be afraid that it will never begin.

—Grace Hansen

So often our focus upon death and the possibility of dying is an escape from our real fear . . . that of living our lives.

We have become comfortable with a way of life that is actually a slow death. Our constant working, busyness, taking care of others, and rushing around relieves us of the responsibility of being fully alive and kills us slowly, and in a socially acceptable way to boot. What more could we ask for?

Why are we so afraid of living our lives? What would our lives be like if we decided to show up for them and live them? Why is it so frightening to anticipate feeling our feelings and being present to each moment?

MY INNER PROCESS never gives me more than I can handle. I may not like handling it, and I *can* handle it. It is when I refuse to handle my life that it backs up on me.

❧ April 3

INTERGENERATIONAL PATTERNS

> *Today we are so busy even our stomachs multi-task. Multi-tasking for multi-symptoms—acid-indigestion, gas pressure, bloating and discomfort, and heartburn. Fast relief for the way we live.*
>
> —Rolaids ad

There it was right there on the TV screen when I was just looking for a program to enjoy. "Fast relief for the way we live. Multi-tasking for multi-symptoms." I had just been talking to some young businesswomen to see what pressures they were experiencing and how their pressures may differ from those of a generation ago, and the word *multi-tasking* came up again and again. And there it was on TV with a medication to take care of it. Quick work!

Their mothers called it balancing a career and a family. Their mother's mother called it being overextended. It sounds pretty much the same to me. We women are caught in the web of trying to do too much. The problem is intergenerational; we were taught the skills to perpetuate the problem by our mothers and grandmothers. And it must be getting worse if a pill has been invented for it.

HOW DO WE break the intergenerational chain? We don't have to do what our mothers and grandmothers did. We can develop new patterns of behaving. And, we may not get a lot of help along the way.

❧ April 4

INTEGRITY/SUCCESS

Integrity is so perishable in the summer months of success.
—Vanessa Redgrave

I wonder, have I let my integrity slip in order to succeed? Have there been times that I was willing to look the other way or take the easy way out in order to avoid conflict or to gain acceptance?

Every day we are offered opportunities to sacrifice our integrity on issues that may be of the utmost importance or on ones that appear insignificant. Without our integrity, there is no way that we can feel good about ourselves. Success and loss of integrity are not synonymous. In fact, true success requires great integrity.

These "little" incidents of integrity slippage eat away at us like termites. How important it is to stop to take a look at the decisions we have made! What a relief it is to know that our valued integrity is there deep within us and that we can reconnect with it at a moment's notice.

CHECKING **for possible slips of integrity allows me to feel better about myself.**

❧ April 5

CONNECTEDNESS

> *The motions and patterns and connections of things*
> *became apparent on a gut level.*
>
> —Robyn Davidson

Each of us has magical moments in our lives when we become aware of the oneness of all things. When that happens, we see the "motions and patterns and connections." A feeling of warmth permeates our being and we heave a sigh of heartfelt relief. We can know the unknowable. We *know* the unknowable.

Yet when we try to share these experiences, we find ourselves inarticulate. In our feeble attempts to describe them, words seem like balls of cotton growing larger and larger as we try to push them out of our mouths. Often, in talking about such an experience, we lose our connection with the experience itself.

I WILL TRUST these profound pauses. And I know that I cannot have them unless I pause.

✥ April 6

FAILURE

> *The clouds gathered together, stood still and watched the river scuttle around the forest floor, crash headlong into haunches of hills with no notion of where it was going, until exhausted, ill and grieving, it slowed to a stop just twenty leagues short of the sea.*
>
> —Toni Morrison

My, can that woman write! I read a passage like the one above, and I just want to read it over and over. It is such a beautiful description of how we sometimes bash and batter ourselves in trying to reach a goal and then end up "ill and grieving" and exhausted, not realizing that we are almost there. We, like the river, rush helter-skelter, headlong into the barriers of our being.

NONE OF US can avoid failure. We *can* avoid battering ourselves in the process.

⁂ April 7

MONOTONE MINDS

Life ought to be a struggle of desire toward adventures whose nobility will fertilize the soul.

—Rebecca West

One of the side effects of doing too much is developing monotone minds. We spend so much time in our work and in work-related activities that our awarenesses and our perceptions become narrower and narrower. We reach a point where we can't talk about anything but our work and, if the truth be known, we don't *want* to talk about anything but our work.

We have become dull and uninteresting. We may even find that we're bored with ourselves. This happens to those of us who work full-time at home, and it happens to those who sit at the top of a corporation.

We have taken a rainbow and compressed it into a solid, uninteresting beam of light.

THE TEARS for myself may be the prism needed to rediscover the rainbow that is me.

❧ April 8

FRIENDSHIP

> *She became for me an island of light, fun, wisdom where I could run with my discoveries and torments and hopes at any time of day and find welcome.*

—May Sarton

We sometimes forget all the friends we have had in our lives. The negative thinking of our disease tends to focus on what is missing. But let's take today and let ourselves remember the friends who have been there for us.

For me, there was the little old lady with the beautiful flower garden who would not let my parents spank me when I tried to pick some flowers and inadvertently pulled them up by the roots. "She was only admiring their beauty," she said when my mother marched me over to apologize. And there was the friend in grade school who came forward to share the rap when I was the only one caught. There were friends who shared our tentative relationships and sexual explorations and never told. There were friends we studied with, hung out with, and grew up with—who were there for us. There were adults who served as models and mentors and judged us not. There were friends.

REMEMBERING the friends I have had in my life caresses my mind and being like a warm bath caresses my body.

❧ April 9

VICTIMS

We cannot have a world where everyone is a victim. "I'm this way because my father made me this way. I'm this way because my husband made me this way." Yes, we are indeed formed by traumas that happen to us. But you must take charge, you must take over, you are responsible.

—Camille Paglia

We live in a world of victims. Modern psychology is victim psychology. Unfortunately, everyone who truly believes she is a victim will become a perpetrator. That's the truth of it. Whether we realize it or not, the moment we admit to being a victim, we want to get someone. Victim psychology creates perpetrators large and small.

Yet there's another way. Many of us have been *victimized* who never became *victims*. We are formed by our traumas *and* it is up to us what we do with the traumatic events that we have experienced.

Instead of moving to victim and then perpetrating, we can admit the trauma, deal with the feelings, get the learnings, and integrate those learnings into becoming a person who is responsible for our lives.

After all, the perpetrator has to deal with what she/he did. That's none of our business. It's our business, however, when we become the perpetrator.

WE CANNOT prevent traumas from happening to us. What we do with them is up to us. The choice of our response will affect the rest of our lives.

❧ April 10

OUR PHYSICAL HEALTH

Toxic ideas—about "a woman's place"; about father knowing best. About the doctor always being right. About drugs and surgery being your only medical options. As you can see, these, if used unnecessarily, can be very dangerous to a woman's physical and emotional health.

—Christiane Northrup

How much time are we willing to give to our physical and emotional health? Often, we expect our bodies to keep humming along with minimum maintenance.

A few years ago I had a gallbladder attack—ouch! The first doctor I went to see, my doctor's personal physician, instantly diagnosed the problem and said, "Immediate surgery!" Through my fog I asked, "What are my other options?"

"None," he said.

"Why none?" I asked.

"That's the quickest solution," he said.

"I have time," I said.

Another told me if I wouldn't have surgery he didn't want to see me again. At least we agreed on that!

I then did my research. Glorious options!—diet, minerals, vitamins, cleanses. Within four months I was symptom and gall stone free. I felt great.

Quick is not always best. We can't be too willing to turn our important decisions over to others for expediency.

WE NEED to give ourselves time to explore options for our physical health. Then we'll know what's best.

BUSYNESS/RUSHING/DISTRACTIBILITY

> *A mark of a true workaholic is cleaning house in your
> underwear.*

> —Coleen

We women who do too much can see so many unfinished projects and so many things that need to be done
that we are easily distracted. Getting dressed in the
morning is not always an easy process. We take our
shower, and then we see something that needs to be
done. We get our underwear on, and then we see something that needs to be done. It is difficult to focus on the
task at hand, and when we do, we see a million other little things that we'll just tidy up before we get dressed.

Surely we have time to pick up the papers on the way
to the kitchen to get our morning coffee. On the way
back to the bathroom we can straighten the pillows on
the couch. If we put the laundry in now, it can run while
we do a quick vacuum.

Is it any wonder that we secretly see ourselves as
incompetent? Even though we get a lot of little tasks
done, we are so distractible that we jump from one task
to another and never have a real feeling of completion.
It is helpful to remember that we are cursed with busyness and distractibility. It is only in recognizing these
behaviors as something we have learned and not truly
who we are that we open ourselves to the possibility of
something new.

TAKE A BREATH, **slow down, and finish something.**

❧ April 12

WEEKENDS/UNSTRUCTURED TIME

I hate weekends. There's no structure. There's no compass. How will I know what to do if I don't have to do it?

—Susan

Weekends are awful for women who do too much. We miss the structure of the workweek. We do not like the lack of schedule, and we feel lost without our work.

To avoid experiencing these feelings, we have developed certain insurance strategies. We bring work home. We schedule our weekend projects and activities so that we almost have the secure feeling of being at work. We panic and go into the office to "pick up some things and tie up some loose ends."

WHAT ARE WE afraid of? . . . ourselves?

❧ April 13

OUR MIRRORS

Mirror, mirror on the wall . . .

                       —Snow White's wicked stepmother

We are surrounded by mirrors. People are like mirrors in our lives. We *need* mirrors in our lives.

We have areas that we know about ourselves that others know about us—our public selves. We have areas we know about ourselves that we keep hidden from others—our private selves. We have areas that others know about us that we don't know about ourselves—our unknown selves. And we have areas about ourselves that are unknown to us and unknown to others—our hidden selves. The latter two can result in some serious blind spots that can cause us some troubles down the line if they haven't already.

Since we are so busy, we rarely take the time to focus on these hidden selves so, luckily, we have "mirrors" that prove to be very efficient.

Remember the old saying that "what we react to in others is all too often a hidden part of ourselves"? Well, there can be some truth to that. If we have a strong reaction to someone, we may want to take the time to look inside to see what is going on with us. Likewise, if we are really attracted by someone, maybe we have some of these qualities, too. Learning our unknowns may be the most important journey we ever take—and fun, too.

OUR "MIRRORS" reflect our blind spots so we can push beyond our present self-knowledge.

❧ April 14

NEGATIVITY

> *Most of the mental chatter in your head is usually nega-*
> *tive and self-critical. It's been proven that these negative*
> *thoughts can, indeed, contribute to muscular tension,*
> *high blood pressure, high cholesterol, even heart disease*
> *and immune weakness.*
>
> —Christiane Northrup

Nag, nag, nag. Grumble, grumble, grumble. Chatter, chatter, chatter. How busy our little minds are! How constant is the committee in our heads! If we put in the hours they do, we would be even more exhausted than we are now.

When did we give them residence permits? Did they get our permission to move in? How in the world did they become so negative about us? Are we really that bad?

Once we realize that while we were un-aware, we appointed this committee in our head, then we can also realize that if we appointed them we have the power to dismiss and fire them. What fun!

**NEGATIVITY is one of the ways we withdraw from our-
selves and others.**

✤ April 15

ACCEPTANCE/HONESTY

With him for a sire and her for a dam,
What should I be but just what I am?
>   —Edna St. Vincent Millay

Some of us do not know the difference between putting ourselves down, thus refusing to accept our gifts and talents, and accepting who we are.

Indeed, we often bounce between being worthless and being totally arrogant. Interestingly, feeling like we are worthless and feeling that we are unique and wonderful are intimately related. In both illusions, we refuse to see ourselves as we really are.

It is only when we are able to say, "I know nothing about that," or "I am really good at doing that and quite knowledgeable about that," that we are moving toward acceptance of self. Seeing our shortcomings allows us to accept them. Accepting our strengths allows us to soar. Honesty about self is the key.

TODAY I have the opportunity not to be grandiose about either my shortcomings or my capabilities. I can be me.

❧ April 16

INDEPENDENCE

> *Dependency invites encroachment.*
> —Patricia Meyer Spacks

We women who do too much are terrified of being dependent. We clearly understand that "dependency invites encroachment." Unfortunately, our fear of dependency often results in behavior that looks like independence but is really what the psychologists call counterdependence. We are so afraid of dependency that we can't trust anyone, which means that we are still controlled by our dependency needs. Whenever we are circling around any form of dependency, whether it be dependence, independence, or interdependence, we probably are in trouble.

Another option is not to define ourselves in terms of dependency. We can learn to be self-defining. We can learn not to ask others to form our identities for us. Only then can we be truly free and bring the gift of ourselves to any relationship.

INDEPENDENCE **and dependence may both be cages.**

✢ April 17

ADVICE GIVING

> *Show me a wife who doesn't offer advice and I'll show you one who doesn't care very much.*
>
> —Barbara Bush

Offering advice has fallen in disrepute as of late. It's not politically correct. Or so we are lead to believe.

Yet, what is a marriage certificate if it isn't a license to offer advice?

Now, let's be careful with this offering advice bit. First of all, offering advice is not telling someone what to do. That's always a bad move with other adults and often even with children.

Good advice offering requires knowing a person very, very well. So well, in fact, that you may know more abut them than they know about themselves in certain situations. Then, good advice is loving and given out of love. It is never to control or manipulate. Then, it is giving information; just giving, not enforcing, information. And lastly and most importantly, after advice is given, the outcome is let go of completely, trusting that the other person will take it, leave it, or ponder it.

ONCE ADVICE, **in the form of information, is given, it is no longer ours.**

❧ April 18

APPRECIATION

And to all those voices of wisdom that have whispered to me along the way.

—Dhyani Ywahoo

Gratitude and appreciation are important facets of our lives. There have been so many women who have shared their wisdom and their knowledge with us. Some of that wisdom has been learned from others, and some of it has been self-taught, and all of it has been profound.

Remember the neighbor who taught us how to care for plants? Remember the mother who shared some helpful hints about staying out of the way of our children? Remember that little old lady in our place of worship who quietly seemed to live what we were being taught about spirituality? Remember that book that seemed just to appear when we needed it? There have been voices of wisdom all around us all our lives.

PERHAPS, as one of my wise friends says, "It's time to have a gratitude attack."

❧ April 19

ADJUSTING

> If we have not achieved our early dreams, we must either
> find new ones or see what we can salvage from the old. If
> we have accomplished what we set out to do in our
> youth, then we need not weep like Alexander the Great
> that we have no worlds to conquer. There is clearly much
> left to be done, and whatever else we are going to do, we
> had better get on with it.
>
> —Roselynn Carter

Life is a series of adjustments, not compromises, because compromises always imply someone losing something and settling for something less than she wanted. If we think in terms of adjustments to constantly changing circumstances, pressures, and realities, we see just how marvelously skilled and talented we are.

We women who do too much often have difficulty with adjustments. We have our lives planned down to the second, and any unexpected change we can view as a personal attack and fight against with "appropriate" vehemence.

Adjustments and the ability to adjust may be the key to making our life easier. When I went to camp in the summer, they repeated a slogan like a mantra—"It's a mark of leadership to adjust." True leaders don't always have to have their way. True leaders may be the ones who have the vision to see what needs to be done and adjust.

ADJUSTING **and getting on with it may save our lives.**

❧ April 20

REALITY/INVENTORY

You need to claim the events of your life to make yourself yours. When you truly possess all you have been and done, which may take some time, you are fierce with reality.

—Flonda Scott Maxwell

Being "fierce with reality" requires that we break through our denial about ourselves and our lives layer by layer. At some point in our lives, we need to stop and take a thorough inventory of who we are and what we have done. This fearless and searching inventory not only focuses upon the things that we have done wrong and the things we wish we had done in some other way, it also focuses upon our strengths and the things we have done right.

So many of us forget that taking stock of ourselves also means writing down what is good about us and the things we appreciate and like about ourselves. After all, honesty is not only about the mistakes, it is also about the good, the powerful, the creative, the loving, and the gentle, compassionate aspects of ourselves.

WHEN WE STOP and truly possess all we have been, and done, we are on the path to becoming who we are.

❧ April 21

SELF-AWARENESS

> *Until the missing story of ourselves is told, nothing besides told can suffice us: we shall go on quietly craving it.*
> —Laura Riding

Probably the most important journey we will ever take is the journey inward. Unless we know who we are, how can we possibly offer what we have?

Each of us is a unique combination of heredity and experiences. No one else has to offer what we have to offer. Yet, if we do not have the self-awareness to undergird our uniqueness, we never make our contribution.

One of the most disastrous effects of our doing too much is that we never really have the time for the process of self-awareness, and then, when we do, we may be too exhausted to care.

I NEED to know my story . . . all of it.

❧ April 22

SELF-RESPECT

When self-respect takes its rightful place in the psyche of woman, she will not allow herself to be manipulated by anyone.

—Indira Mahindra

Being a woman isn't always the easiest thing in the world, but it's what I have to work with right now. There are so many aspects of ourselves that merit self-respect. We are unbelievably competent at what we do. We are flexible and strong and can be both simultaneously. We have good ideas that are practical and creative, and we can articulate them well. We have the ability to deal with several tasks simultaneously and attend to each one. We are organizers, creators, and doers and we have a great capacity for being. We have much to contribute including a perspective on life that is different from that of the men around us. We are here to stay, and we and others need to accept that fact.

MY SELF-RESPECT is not only essential to me, it is important to the world.

❧ April 23

GUILT

> *Shit work is infinitely safe. In exchange for doing it you can extract an unconscionable return . . . the women's pound of flesh.*
>
> —Colette Dowling

We are often experts in guilt. Certainly we have learned it from masters. We unquestionably and with great doggedness go about our assigned tasks without a grumble or a reproach.

We are armed, however, with our sighs, our clenched teeth, our pathetic looks of acceptance, and our sagging shoulders. Our favorite phrase is "That's okay," but we really don't mean it. One of our greatest skills is suffering, and we do it so well. We get our pound of flesh, and we lose our souls in the process.

TELL ME, is it really worth it? Are we ready to give up the guilt game? It gets infinitely boring.

❧ April 24

BEING PROJECTLESS

Out of the strain of the Doing,
Into the peace of the Done.

—Julia Louise Woodruff

When most women finish a task, they heave a sigh of relief, pat themselves on the back, and give themselves a well-deserved break. Not so for women who do too much. The "peace of the Done" simply does not compute. There is no experience to which we can relate this concept.

Fortunately, as we let ourselves see that we are not just talking about doing too much, we begin to have a different perspective.

We begin to learn that completion and beginning are not the same process. We begin to see that the completion of an important project has every right to be dignified by a natural grieving process. Something that required the best of us has ended. We will miss it.

BEING PROJECTLESS **and being worthless are not synonymous.**

✺ April 25

BELIEF

The experience of God, or in any case the possibility of experiencing God, is innate.

—Alice Walker

We cry to a God "out there," and our voices return like burned-out spaceships that have traversed the universe. We ask authorities how to experience God and realize that they have come to worship their rituals and techniques, yet seem to know little of God. No ancient prophet lost in the wilderness felt more isolated than we do as we buzz around the wilderness of our cities and organizations. How could any God get through this steel and concrete?

Yet, when we stop, we have a glimmer of understanding of what it means to say that "the possibility of experiencing God is innate." We do not have to look for that possibility. It is already in us.

THE POSSIBILITY of experiencing a power greater than myself has always been there, knocking on my inner door.

❧ April 26

BUSYNESS

The season is changeable, fitful, and maddening as I am myself these days that are cloaked with too many demands and engagements.

—May Sarton

When we do not recognize that we have become too busy and overextended, we too find ourselves being "changeable, fitful, and maddening." Our lack of awareness of our needs and our inability to attend to them sets up a situation where our only recourse is to become so obnoxious that others will leave us alone. Then we do not have to take the responsibility for stating that we need time to ourselves and taking it. Of course, this particular technique for getting alone time usually results in fences that need to be mended.

There are other ways of having what we need. We can let ourselves know that we need time to ourselves and then we can arrange to have it.

TAKING THE TIME I need for myself when I need it may be a lot less exciting than creating a crisis, and it certainly is less messy.

❧ April 27

CHOICES/FEELING TRAPPED

> *I discovered I always have choices and sometimes it's only a choice of attitude.*
>
> —Judith M. Knowlton

One of the most devastating characteristics of our doing-too-much process is that our perceptions, our judgment, and our thinking become so distorted that we come to believe that we have no choices and are completely trapped. We have the illusion that there are only two choices (usually to stay or leave) and neither looks attractive.

We do have options. We do have choices, even if the only choice available at the moment is to see that we are stuck and to accept that "stuckness." Amazingly, when we truly accept our stuckness, our situations begin to change. Often it is not the situation that is keeping us stuck but our *attitude* about our situation.

CHOICES are part of being human. When I feel I have no choices, I am probably operating out of my disease.

❧ April 28

BEAUTY

> *Oh, it was a glorious morning! I suppose the best kind of spring morning is the best weather God has to offer. It certainly helps one to believe in Him [sic].*
>
> —Dodie Smith

How long has it been since we have allowed ourselves to rejoice in a beautiful day? How long has it been since we allowed ourselves to notice that it even is a beautiful day?

Those of us who live and work in cities have given ourselves obstacles that challenge us to have to work a little harder even to notice what kind of day it is.

For women who do too much, the beautiful day may be noteworthy only in the absence of hassle that rain or snow might present. A beautiful day, then, only becomes the vehicle to get more done. There are other options.

I LONG for the awareness to say, "Oh, it was a glorious morning!"

❧ April 29

FEAR/MANIPULATION

> *All women hustle. Women watch faces, voices, gestures,*
> *moods. The person who has to survive through cunning.*
> —Marge Piercy

Most women are accomplished research scientists. We have developed skills for gathering data that would put most researchers to shame. We are constantly scanning faces, bodies, and situations for clues about what is acceptable and what we can get away with. We have, unfortunately, in many situations become people who "survive through cunning." Our hyperalertness emanates from our fear that whatever we do will not be enough—our fear that *we* are not enough no matter what we do. We have to be cunning to survive, or so we have come to believe. We scan and hustle and we don't even know we are doing it.

I AM ENOUGH. **We all will just have to accept what I have to give.**

❧ April 30

ISOLATION

> *One of the reasons our society has become such a mess is that we're isolated from each other.*
>
> —Maggie Kuhn

Isolation is one of the characteristics of women who do too much.

We may be surrounded by people all day long, but our singleminded dedication to our work and our rushing isolates us. We do not like to be interrupted by friends. We would rather get our work done. We get angry when things don't fall into place and others are afraid to approach us.

We have become just as locked up and closeted with our working, our busyness, our hurrying around as our grandmothers were in their isolated houses. We have forgotten how to reach out, and we don't have the time for it, even if we remember how. We think if we just had more time to focus on our work we'd feel better, and instead we feel exhausted. Isolation is an energy drain.

I NEED to learn the difference between isolation and solitude.

❧ May 1

> *Normal day, let me be aware of the treasure you are. Let me learn from you, love you, bless you before you depart. Let me not pass you by in quest of some rare and perfect tomorrow. Let me hold you while I may, for it may not always be so. One day I shall dig my nails into the earth, or bury my face in the pillow, or stretch myself taut, or raise my hands to the sky and want, more than all the world, your return.*

—Mary Jean Iron

This moment is right now. It is what we have. How often we have squandered the treasure of today and dreamed of the fortunes of the future, only to mourn for the loss of this day. Today, we can see the excitement in the eyes of a child over some new discovery. Today, we can listen to an old friend before we get on to the next task. Have we missed today by not being present to it? Will we later weep tears of mourning and wish for its return? How much better to live it today.

JUST **a normal day—what a gift!**

❧ May 2

COURAGE

Remember, Ginger Rogers did everything Fred Astaire did, but she did it backwards and in high heels.

—Faith Whittlesey

That's right! Ginger Rogers was amazingly good at what she did, and so are we. It takes courage for women to acknowledge how good we are at what we do. We are caught in a strange cultural expectation of having to be simultaneously competent and passive. This often results in a kind of humility that really is a denial of our expertise.

Also, women who do too much seem to vacillate between exaggerating our competence and feeling that we are worthless and totally incompetent. This vacillation between extremes is part of the whole syndrome of doing too much.

The real test of courage is being realistic and letting ourselves know that we really are competent at many things.

BEING GOOD at what we do isn't a curse. It's a gift that comes from ourselves *and* from a power greater than ourselves.

❧ May 3

DESPAIR

That was a time when only the dead could smile.

—Anna Akhmatova

We have known times like these. In fact, the point where we realized that we had to admit that doing too much was no longer something that *we* did, it did us, and was our personal moment of hitting bottom. Before we completely admitted our powerlessness over our working too much, we despaired, fearing that nothing could change.

Yet we *have* changed. We have reached the depths of despair and lived through it. We have gone into the abyss and found that God is nothingness too.

We remember our despair, and we are also grateful to it, because hitting bottom has paved the way for new ways of being, and that's great.

THE GOOD THING about reaching a point of despair is that it has opened up a possibility of a whole new life for me.

❧ May 4

LIVING IN THE PRESENT

Yesterday is a cancelled check
Tomorrow is a promissory note
Today is cash in hand; spend it wisely.

—Anonymous

What a challenge to live in the present! We are often so busy killing the present moment with worries about tomorrow or regrets about yesterday that we kill our todays. Ironically, all we can really do is be in the present.

Living in the present means noticing—noticing when we are tired, noticing when we need to go the bathroom, noticing when we need to rest.

Living in the present means taking a walk for the sake of the walk, not just to get someplace. Living in the present means noticing and appreciating our now. Living in the present means doing our lives, not thinking about them.

IF I DO MY LIFE then I won't be undone.

❧ May 5

FEELING OVERWHELMED

> *The social workers have named a new syndrome. It's called "compassion fatigue." Why does it sound so familiar?*
> —Anne Wilson Schaef

Careaholics never quite know when it all happened. We were trained to believe that, if we just took care of people and listened and understood, they in turn would take care of us. We firmly believed that relationships are built on people taking care of each other, and if we took care first, we would certainly get the same in return. What a shock to find out that this belief is not only not held by everyone, but the more we take care of people, the more they want.

We feel drained, resentful, taken advantage of, and overwhelmed. Those seem to be normal feelings in the situation. Thank goodness we don't have to stay stuck there, however. Just recognizing the feelings helps us begin to check out our assumptions about caretaking.

LOVING isn't caretaking and caretaking isn't love. We can't buy love . . . it's a gift.

❧ May 6

WOMEN'S PERCEPTIONS

> *An English professor wrote on the blackboard—*
> *"Woman without her man is a savage." The students*
> *were instructed to punctuate it correctly. Men wrote,*
> *"Woman, without her man, is a savage." Women wrote,*
> *"Woman: without her, man is a savage."*
>
> —Anonymous

Ah perceptions—differing perceptions. I wonder if one of the reasons women do too much is because, historically, our perceptions of reality have been ignored—or labeled "crazy"?

We work hard to prove that we can and do perceive the accepted-majority reality accurately.

We work hard to ignore and sublimate our own perceptions.

We work hard not to let it matter that we have to develop a whole new group of perceptions to be acceptable and "get ahead."

We work hard to ignore the feelings that come up in us when our perceptions are ignored or ridiculed.

It's a lot of work to work so hard.

THE WORLD **desperately needs women's perceptions of reality.**

UNWRAPPING TO US

If you're all wrapped up in yourself, you're overdressed.
—Kate Halverson

It's difficult to be overdressed in today's styles, isn't it? And, we can be so full of ourselves that it doesn't matter what we do or how we do it, we're often too much for ourselves and others.

Women have neglected ourselves for so many centuries that it seems that some of us are trying to make up for centuries of neglect. In the process, we may go overboard and become self-centered and self-seeking. It's not a pretty sight.

We haven't had much practice with the subtle nuances between taking care of ourselves and being self-centered. Indeed, thanks to the "me" generation and lots of New Age fodder, we have come to believe that taking care of ourselves means always putting "me" first, pushing in ahead of others, driving aggressively, and generally being all wrapped up in ourselves.

Not so! In fact, when we are self-centered we are usually completely out of touch with ourselves. We are running on automatic and, often, not in touch with what's really important to us. Our head and our distorted beliefs are dictating our thoughts and behavior, while our essence is left somewhere in the dust.

IT'S TIME to get back in touch with that many-faceted person underneath those camouflages. She'll know what to do.

❧ May 8

SERENITY

> *She would greet us pleasantly, and immediately she seemed to surround the chaotic atmosphere of morning strife with something of order, of efficient and quiet uniformity, so that one had the feeling that life was small and curiously ordered.*
>
> —Meridel LeSueur

Whew! Isn't it a relief to know that there are people in the world who are so present to the moment that when they enter a chaotic atmosphere they create calm? This calm is not born of control or manipulation. This calm is born of presence.

Only a person who is present to herself carries a feeling of serenity with her. Hopefully we can begin to experience this kind of serenity for ourselves.

ORDER that comes out of control is full of tension. Order that comes out of rigidity is full of strife. Order that comes out of serenity is peaceful.

✣ May 9

BUSYNESS/LONELINESS

You can get lonesome—being that busy.

—Isabel Lennart

Workaholics are lonely people. Our work is like a jealous lover. It demands more and more of us. We see ourselves becoming progressively isolated from those who are important to us. We schedule lunches two weeks in advance so that we can keep up social contact with friends and then have to break or postpone these lunches because "something has come up." We get "antsy" if we are interrupted; we get irritable if someone stops by to talk because we want to get back to our work. We often don't know we are lonely because we don't stop long enough to let ourselves know what we are feeling.

IT IS GOOD to be productive, and busyness is no substitute for intimacy.

❧ May 10

INTIMACY

So instant intimacy was too often followed by disillusion.
—May Sarton

We live in an age of instant dinners, instant success, and instant intimacy. We expect ourselves to meet someone and know immediately that we were meant for each other. After all, in our busy lives we don't have the time for long, drawn-out courtships.

Instant intimacy is one of the characteristics of dysfunctional relationships. In fact, when clear women experience a bit of instant intimacy, they have learned to run for the hills. This kind of instant connection usually does not wear well.

Intimacy takes time. It is a process. It needs to be fed, valued, nurtured, and allowed to grow. When we try to manipulate intimacy, we kill it. In fact, we often use instant intimacy to avoid the possibility of real intimacy.

INTIMACY takes time. If I don't have time, I probably won't have intimacy.

❧ May 11

ANGUISH

Each woman is being made to feel it is her own cross to bear if she can't be the perfect clone of the male superman and the perfect clone of the feminine mystique.

—Betty Friedan

No wonder we sometimes find ourselves filled with anguish. There is just too much to do. Too many demands are made upon us. We are asked to be too many people—some of whom we are and some of whom we are not. Anguish is probably a normal response to such a situation.

Luckily, we do not have to stop with anguish. It is important to feel our anguish, go through it, and move on. One of the ways we stay stuck is to block our feelings and refuse to admit them. Sometimes life presents us with vises, puts us in them, and screws them tight. Then we find that as we let ourselves feel our feelings of hurt and anguish, we can move on.

WHEN WE admit that feeling anguish could very possibly be normal in our situation, we're on our way.

LOVE

> *I wish I'd a knowed more people. I would of loved 'em all. If I'd a knowed more, I woulda loved more.*
>
> —Toni Morrison

We all have an infinite capacity for loving. Sometimes we get confused about loving, and we start thinking that we only have so much to go around. We start thinking in zero-sum terms. We believe that we only have so much love and if we give some away, we have that much less. We start parceling out our love like we pay the bills at the end of the month. We meet all of our "love obligations," and we try to keep a little bit in savings, just in case of an emergency. Controlled love is not loving. Obligatory love is not loving. Love is something that flows out of our deep sense of loving ourselves. It is not possible to love another if we don't know and love ourselves.

When we love ourselves, there is no limit to the amount of love we can share. But loving can never be manufactured because we should, need to, or want to get something in return. Love is an energy that is shared because we have it.

LOVING the people I know allows me to know the people I love.

❧ May 13

PARENTING

The thing about having a baby is that thereafter you have it.

—Jean Kerr

What a shock! Our children do not always fit into our fantasies. They do not always provide us with the "perfect little family." They do not always fit in with our schemes and plans. And the worst thing about them is that we simply cannot get them shaped up the way we want them and expect them to stay that way.

When we give birth to a child, we give birth to a process that continues in one form or another for the rest of our lives. Somehow, we seemed to have missed the concept that parenting is an intimate interactive process that continues.

WHEN WE STOP trying to make our children fit our fantasies of who they *should* be, we can begin to see who they are!

RESPONSIBILITY/GUILT

If you believe you are to blame for everything that goes wrong, you are going to stay until you fix it.

—Susan Forward

We women who do too much are *responsible.* That is one of our great virtues, or so we think. We are willing to take accountability and blame for *everything.* When something happens at work, it must be our fault. If our relationships fail, we must have done something wrong. If our children have difficulties, we are to blame. Guilt and blame are old familiar friends. It is inconceivable to us that we did not cause . . . whatever. This is one form of our self-centeredness. We put ourselves right squarely in the middle of any disaster. Of course, the other side of the dualism is to be totally blameless and a victim. We bounce back and forth between the two.

What a difference it is to move into respondability, a place where accountability and blame have no meaning and our ability to respond is the key.

MY ABILITY to respond is hampered by accountability and blame.

TAKING OUR PLACE

The ceiling isn't glass; it is a very dense layer of men.
—Anne Jardim

Who invented the idea of the glass ceiling anyway? We were supposed to be able to see through it but we could never penetrate it—right? Hmmm. Do we really see through it? Are we really privy to what is actually going on at the highest levels of business and politics in our world? I doubt it. Do we want to be?

Do we want the responsibility to make the decisions that affect ourselves and the world around us on a daily basis? Do we just keep as busy as we can so we don't have to answer or even consider the hard places? Would we rather stay dumb, irresponsible, and grumble? I don't think so. We want a future. We want a future for our children. We want a future for our parents. We care about the decisions being made above the glass ceiling.

At some point, we strong, beautiful, caring, intelligent, and brave women need to step back and see what our doing too much is keeping us from *not* doing. We may be shocked.

HOW LONG have we been willing to let men carry the load?

❧ May 16

ASKING FOR HELP

Advice is what we ask for when we already know the answer but wish we didn't.

—Erica Jong

Right! Usually when we ask for advice, it is because we are already aware of the answer within us, and we do not want to heed our inner knowing. Let someone else take the rap!

Also, when we ask for advice, there is a part of us just daring anyone to give it. When they do, it takes the pressure off of us, even when we know it will not work and we will secretly reject it.

Asking for help, on the other hand, is a completely different matter. Most women who do too much have great difficulty asking for help. We usually can do it ourselves, whatever "it" is, and are more comfortable doing it ourselves. We can give orders and *tell* others to do what needs to be done. We can organize and supervise. We have learned many ways of getting help without asking for it and without admitting we need it. Yet, there is something infinitely more honest in asking for help when we need it.

ASKING FOR HELP does not mean that we are weak or incompetent. It usually indicates an advanced level of honesty and intelligence.

✶ May 17

AWARENESS

> *I felt like I was in a fog. I knew that I was desperately*
> *searching for something of great importance, the loss of*
> *which was life-threatening, but I couldn't see clearly.*
>
> —Judy Ness

We keep ourselves so busy and so overworked that we do not have time to see that we are in a fog and searching for something of great importance.

We look to our work, our money, or our families to fulfill us, and all these "solutions" fail miserably.

Even if we are successful, when we stop long enough we are aware of a feeling of loneliness and emptiness. We have failed to realize that nothing from outside can really fill us up and that the person we really long to find is ourselves. Not having ourselves and not being in touch with ourselves is life-threatening. When we leave ourselves, we are more vulnerable to outside influences and less aware of what we really need.

How exciting it is to begin to see the fog lift and to know that that for which we so desperately search has been there within us all the time.

WHAT I am looking for is not "out there." It is in me. It is me.

TALENTS

> *When I stand before God at the end of my life, I would
> hope that I would not have a single bit of talent left and
> could say, "I used everything you gave me."*
>
> —Erma Bombeck

One of my favorite Bible stories was the story of the
talents. God gave one person one talent and he (of
course, "he") went away and developed it and used it
and God was pleased. To another, God gave many talents and he went away and squandered them and God
was not pleased. Well, I sure wanted to please God, and
I went about developing and using my talents, which
appeared to be quite a bunch.

Then, when I was a young mother, working full-time,
making all my daughter's clothes (and mine and my
husband's sports jackets!), cooking, singing in the choir,
. . . and, and, and, I became exhausted. Upon reflection
and reconsideration, I decided I wanted to do the best I
could by God and that the generosity of God's gifts
meant that I simply could not spend them all and might
have to pick and choose a bit. I miss some of my talents
that are going unspent, and doing what I can and need
to do seems enough.

Maybe the issue is not the compulsive spending of
talents. It is the use of my talents to live and serve as fully
as I can.

BEING COMPULSIVE about the gifts we have been given
doesn't work. Using them enough works just fine.

❧ May 19
RELATING TO MEN

One of the things about equality is not just that you be treated equally to a man, but that you treat yourself equally to the way you treat a man.

—Marlo Thomas

Aha! This is a good one to consider. How do we treat men? Do we treat them differently than we treat women? Do we treat them differently than we treat ourselves?

If so, how, when, why? What can we learn about ourselves by taking some time to stand outside ourselves and observe—really observe—the way we treat men to see if there is any difference between the way we treat them, other women, and ourselves. Do I defer? Do I compete? Do I compare? All of these are interesting and important questions.

This is one of the most exciting things we can do in life—to become aware of something, gather some information about it, and use that information to move to a new level of growth and awareness.

When we do too much, we don't take the time for these gigantic leaps in growth and awareness.

TODAY, I have the opportunity to observe how I relate to men and to see if it differs from the way I relate to women and myself. Then, I can see what comes next.

BEING PRESENT TO THE MOMENT

Nobility of character manifests itself at loopholes when it is not provided with large doors.

—Mary Wilkins Freeman

Opportunities do not always come at the time or in the form we had hoped. Instead of blinding flashes of light, they are often still small voices that whisper to us in unexpected moments.

Our potential for greatness is linked with our ability to be present to the moment. Noticing may be one of the most important skills we have. When we are present to notice a small, obscure opportunity, we may discover that we have taken a major turn on the path of our life.

ANYBODY can walk through a wide-open door. I hope for the nobility of character to see the loophole.

❧ May 21

CONFLICT

It's better to be a lion for a day than a sheep all your life.
—Elizabeth Henry

Conflict is inevitable in our lives. We feel conflicted over a choice we must make, and the conflict is within. We feel strongly about the way a business decision must go, and we are in conflict with our peers.

Some of us believe that there are only two options when conflict arises. We must either roar like a lion and impose our will or back off like a sheep and give in (and *subtly* try to impose our will). Neither choice has much to say for it.

Thank goodness we have another option. We can check out what is going on inside of us. We can listen to what others are saying. We can get clear with ourselves and see what we have to learn.

CONFLICT **is inevitable. Fighting is a choice.**

❧ May 22

CONNECTEDNESS/CONFUSION/LONELINESS

Women who set a low value on themselves make life hard for all women.

—Nellie McClung

As women we have a special connectedness with each other. We have been raised to be competitive with other women and to see them as enemies and competitors. We have also been raised to see female as inferior and told that if we wanted to get ahead, we needed to identify with men and either become like them or be what they wanted us to be. It has all been very confusing. Frequently, we have felt alone and isolated.

A major factor in our healing has been to recognize that we are women and to seek connectedness with other women. We find ourselves reflected in their stories, and our loneliness changes to connectedness.

I AM NOT ALONE. **Other women share my experiences. Healing and connectedness are the same.**

✿ May 23

CONTROL/ARROGANCE

The passion for setting people right is in itself an afflictive disease.

—Marianne Moore

Women who do too much often think that it is our job to set others right. After much gathering of information and acquisition of knowledge, we really have come to believe that we can and do know what is best for other people. Since we know what is best, we have no difficulty sharing this important information with any who will—or sometimes even will not—listen. Some of us even get *paid* for knowing what is best for others and setting them right.

Ugh, it doesn't look so good on paper, does it?

PERHAPS TODAY would be a good day to look at my arrogance. Benevolent arrogance is still arrogance.

❧ May 24

HOPES AND DREAMS

> *As long as we think dugout canoes are the only possibility—all that is real or can be real—we will never see the ship, we will never feel the wind blow.*
>
> —Sonia Johnson

Women who do too much have grown afraid to dream. We know how to lust—after power, after money, after security, after relationships—but we have forgotten how to dream.

Dreaming is not limited to the unreal. Dreaming is stretching the real beyond the limits of the present. Dreaming is not being bound by the merely possible. Dreaming is not safe for our illusion of control and it is infinitely safe for our soul.

When we deprive ourselves of our hopes and dreams, we relegate ourselves to keeping our eyes to the ground, carefully calculating every step, and missing the pictures in the clouds and the double rainbows.

TO HOPE **and dream is not to ignore the practical. It is to dress it in colors and rainbows.**

HEALING

> *The human heart does not stay away too long from that*
> *which hurt it most. There is a return journey to anguish*
> *that few of us are released from making.*
>
> —Lillian Smith

Those hurts and pains that we experience in childhood don't just magically evaporate as we grow older. They rumble around in us, and when we have reached a level of strength, maturity, insight, and awareness to handle them, they come up to be worked through. This is one of the ways our inner being is loving to us. It gives us every opportunity to heal the hurts that we need to heal, and it gives us that opportunity when we are strong enough to handle it.

Frequently, as children, we have experiences that we simply aren't strong enough to handle without a lot of support and help, and often that support is absent. So we push them down and we wait. When we are ready, they come back up. This gives us the chance to work through these old anguishes when we have what we need for this task.

WHEN I AM READY, I will have the opportunity to make these journeys to old hurts with the knowledge that I can heal them and move on.

✤ May 26

LIVING LIFE FULLY

> *And reach for our lives . . . for all life . . . deep into the cosmos that is our own souls.*
>
> —Sonia Johnson

Each of us is a cosmos unto ourselves. When we are living our lives fully, we are separate persons, and we are also one with the universe. We are ourselves with our boundaries, and we are also connected with all things.

Luckily, we are not really asked to live any one else's life. All we have to do is live our own, and that seems to be quite enough for us.

When we live life fully, we allow ourselves to taste the range of our experiences. We see what we see, feel what we feel, and know what we know. We accept every opportunity to live out of our own souls.

LUCKILY, **living life fully is not a task. It is an opportunity.**

❧ May 27

AWARENESS OF PROCESS

> *He was teaching me something about flow, about choosing the right moment for everything, about enjoying the present.*

> —Robyn Davidson

Sometimes our teachers appear in the most unlikely forms. Robyn Davidson is speaking of an old Aborigine who traveled with her for a while. Although their cultures were vastly different, he taught her some elemental wisdom that needed to be acknowledged and experienced in her culture.

We all need to know about flow. Nothing gets done at once even when we demand it. Work and living flow in a series of nonlinear events.

Timing is also very important. We cannot correct and edit a report until it is written. When our boss is having a bad day, it is not a good idea to bring up an interpersonal problem that happened last week. We cannot control another's reactions by choosing "the right moment," and we can choose the time that is best for us. And we always have the choice to stop and enjoy the present.

WHEN I STAY in my present, I have the opportunity to experience the flow of my life.

❧ May 28

BUSYNESS/EXHAUSTION/SLEEP

I am so keyed up I can't go to sleep at night. I just can't relax. I'm lucky if I get five hours of sleep a night.

—Barbie

One of the side effects of our lives as women who do too much is that we get ourselves so keyed up that we cannot get the rest and sleep we so desperately need. We are constantly on the run. Even when our bodies are ready to drop from exhaustion, we cannot relax and let them experience the soothing regeneration of deep sleep. Sometimes, even when we try to let down, it is too painful to let go, and we find we cannot. We are deprived of the healing that occurs in the alpha phase of sleep. We travel on nerves worn ragged like socks that have not been mended by caring hands. We have deprived ourselves of the unconscious experience of pulling together the tattered and torn threads of our souls and reweaving the holes gouged out by the civility of daily skirmishes. We need our rest.

SLEEP is one of the regenerative gifts of life. I only miss it when I don't have it.

❧ May 29

GRATITUDE FOR HAVING LOVED

> *I still miss those I loved who are no longer with me, but I find I am grateful for having loved them. The gratitude has finally conquered the loss.*

> —Rita Mae Brown

How sweet is the taste of lost loves, whether by death or circumstances! Sometimes we are so busy that we never take the time to savor the pure joy of having loved.

A long time ago, one of the great loves of my life and I decided to part because our lives were moving in different directions. There was never any doubt about our loving—just our directions.

Many years later, when I was making my amends to those I had harmed, I wrote him a long letter to apologize for all the things I had handled badly (which were many!). After some time he responded in his usual loving fashion. I had hoped that we could be friends—I could get to know his wife, and our children could know one another. No such luck; his wife would have none of it. Yet, I have never regretted the loving and "the gratitude has finally conquered the loss."

What an honor to have loved everyone I have loved in my life, and there are many in many ways. The gratitude far outweighs the loss.

TODAY, we have the possibility to be grateful for having loved all those we have loved in our life.

FORGIVENESS

Life is filled with the necessity for forgiveness.
—Hillary Rodham Clinton

Like Hillary, we all have the necessity for forgiveness. There is not one woman on this planet who hasn't been faced with the option of holding on to old hurts and resentments or moving into forgiveness.

It is important to remember that forgiveness is not an event. Forgiveness is a process.

First comes the hurt and the anger. I happen to believe that it is important to give our hurt and anger their due. If we don't, they will just go underground and secretly smolder. Forgiving too soon can result in a "head" forgiveness, which counts for nothing. There is absolutely no problem with going into our anger and pain full speed—unless, of course, you plan to hold on to it, savor it, enjoy it, and indulge.

Then, move on. Take the time to work through the feelings and heal. Working through feelings and healing can never be done on a schedule. While we are going through this process, we can let others know that we want to forgive and we're not there yet. We need to respect ourselves.

If we honor our process of hurt, anger, and healing, one day, without our even realizing it, we will feel like we have stepped out of a dark tunnel into the light and we will have forgiven.

EVEN WHEN **I want to, I cannot rush my forgiveness.**

❧ May 31

ACCOMPLISHMENTS

> *I feel very comfortable in what I'm doing, and I'm accomplishing something, and that's important.*
>
> —Roselynn Carter

How wonderful it is to feel comfortable with what we are doing! No fuss, no muss—just feeling comfortable. Realizing that wherever life has placed us we can accomplish something and that it is in the accomplishing something in whatever setting one finds oneself that comfort and serenity emerge.

Perhaps we had dreamy notions about who we would be, where we would be, and what we would accomplish. Dreams are great—as long as they do not remove us from our reality. When we use our dreams that way, we lose! We imagined ourselves with lots of children, and we could only have one. We imagined ourselves as a doctor, and we work in a store. We imagined a big house and an easy life, and both of us have to work to make ends meet. We imagined a lifelong partner, and we have none—oh, well.

How much serenity comes from accepting life on life's terms. Then, we can look around us, see what is there, and make our contribution—our full contribution with what we have available. That's accomplishing something.

OUR GREATEST achievement may be to be comfortable with what we are doing and to accomplish something.

❧ June 1

FREEDOM

We have not owned our freedom long enough to know exactly how it should be used.

—Phyllis McGinley

As we women have struggled to become free, we have tried out various forms of freedom. We used to think we were free when we were the kind of women men wanted us to be. Then we thought we were free when we could be like men. We thought we were free when we could treat men the way we had been treated.

We thought we were free when we had access to jobs where we could reduce our life span through stress-related diseases. We thought we were free when we had made the team and were allowed to play games in which we had no interest. We thought we were free when we had money, power, and influence.

IT TAKES TIME to grow into freedom. We have time yet.

✥ June 2

KEEPING OTHERS DOWN

As long as you keep a person down, some part of you has to be down there to hold him down, so it means you cannot soar as you otherwise might.

—Marion Anderson

Interesting thought, isn't it? When we keep someone—anyone—down, we have to put time, energy, and effort into keeping them there. We may not even be aware of the drain we are putting on ourselves. It can be anyone we are keeping down—an employee, a boss, a neighbor, a friend, an enemy, a child, a husband, our parents—anyone. And, we can be keeping them down in subtle and not-so-subtle ways—not knowing their differences, not recognizing their potential, gossiping about them, believing they are inferior, not as smart as we are, not as creative, not as loving, not as savvy—the list of possibilities goes on and on. In fact, we can be very creative and devious in the way we keep others down. We can even do it with groups of people, usually those unlike us.

Whoever it is and in whatever ways we do it, this whole process of keeping others down costs us greatly. Is it worth it? I doubt it. Can we change this behavior? You bet!

ONE OF THE BEAUTIFUL things about being human is that we can use new information and change ourselves in ways that give us more possibilities for soaring. I don't need to use my energy to keep others down.

❧ June 3

EXHAUSTION

You white people are so strange. We think it is very primitive for a child to have only two parents.

—Australian Aboriginal Elder

Past generations had the luxury and support of extended families. Grandparents were around and often found meaning in sharing stories about their life and times. As children sat listening, their parents felt the warm glow of recognition and familiarity and chuckled inwardly as old tales were told and retold.

But now many of us are isolated from extended family, or we don't have the time for family. We are it for our children. We have to be past, present, and guides to the future. This is exhausting.

OUR CHILDREN still need to hear the "family stories." So do we.

❧ June 4

GOALS

We were brought up with the value that as we sow, so shall we reap. We discarded the idea that anything we did was its own reward.

—Janet Harris

We live in a goal-oriented society. We are often so busy trying to get to the top of the mountain that we forget to notice the rocks with lichen, the alpine flowers, and even the people along the way. We are ruled by the cult of the orgasm. Foreplay is only a means to an end. Yet for many women the touching, holding, talking, stroking, and intimacy are equally if not more important that the moment of orgasm. Orgasms and goals can be fun, but not if they obliterate everything that goes before.

Setting goals can be useful and important, especially if we are willing to let them go when they become irrelevant, and if we remember that the journey itself is important.

IF I LOOK only at the top of the mountain, I may miss the fossils along the mountainside that can teach me about time and my place in the universe.

❧ June 5

Being in Charge

Never retract, never explain, never apologize . . . get the thing done and let them howl.

—Nellie McClery

There are so many levels on which one could respond to this quote. At one level, it sounds like advice on how to be a bulldozer and run down anyone who offers opposition. I don't recommend that.

At another level, one can zero in on the time lost in explaining, retracting, and apologizing, while the house is burning down. There is something to be said for just moving ahead.

And at another level, when we clearly feel the direction we must take and the job we must get done, there is a certain serenity that emerges when we are truly willing to "let them howl."

HOW WONDERFUL that every issue has so many levels of truth. That makes life anything but dull.

BELIEF

> *I'll bet you when you get down on them rusty knees and get to worrying God, He goes in his privy-house and slams the door. That's what he thinks about you and your prayers.*

—Zora Neale Hurston

Many of us who do too much have long since forsaken our childhood "God" and have found nothing to replace "Him." When we have called upon "Him," we were sure that he went "in his privy-house" and slammed the door. The sound of that door slamming has echoed and careened throughout our aloneness. We were on our own now. We had to do it ourselves. How dualistic we have been. If the God of our childhood didn't work, we would have no contact with any spirituality. Yet, the real loss is our loss of contact with our spiritual selves. We do need time for prayer, meditation, and reflection that is congruent with who we are. When we take that time, we find there is something there beyond ourselves.

BELIEF is not always easy for me. Most of all, my thinking gets in the way.

❧ June 7

SHIFTING PERCEPTIONS

Your worst humiliation is only someone else's momentary entertainment.

—Karen Crockett

Come on now. It's all right that God created human beings for amusement and entertainment. That idea even amuses us. But our humiliations being other people's entertainment? We'll have to think long and hard about that one.

Yet, actually this humiliation-entertainment thing might not be a bad idea after all. It sort of takes the sting out of humiliations, doesn't it?

If we just sit a bit and think about past humiliations, we can find a bit of humor in every one of them by just shifting our perceptions ever so slightly.

In fact, if we just think of the loving teasing we have experienced over the years, we were always able to be amusing to someone. We don't have to see it as at our expense. We really are much more entertaining than we had realized.

WHEN WE **shift our perception ever so slightly, new possibilities always appear.**

❧ June 8

CLUTTER

> *Clutter is what silts up exactly like silt in a flowing stream when the current, the free flow of the mind, is held up by an obstruction.*
>
> —May Sarton

Clutter seems like a constant in our lives. Our houses are cluttered, our desks are cluttered, our minds are cluttered, and our lives are cluttered. This is the curse of women who do too much.

We can never find our creative selves unless we reduce some of the clutter in our lives. The mind must have the opportunity to flow freely if we are to be healthy.

We are such strong, powerful, beautiful, and intelligent women. The world needs what we have to offer.

WE HAVE so many forms of clutter in our lives. We may need to simplify.

❧ June 9

SOLUTIONS

> *The ugly scapegoating that divides our country is the problem, not the solution.*
>
> —Barbara Bush

Part of a frantic lifestyle is that we start to get our identity through the problems we face and begin to place our focus on the problems.

Now, let's don't sell ourselves short. We women who do too much are great with problems. We can tackle problems that no faint heart would even look at. If the truth be known, we love problems. We shine when there are problems. We love the adrenaline rush as we face into a big one. We get a reputation for dealing with problems. We come to identify with problems.

But what about the solution? The solutions are often not nearly as exciting as the problems. Solutions usually require a slowing down, a reconsidering, a compromise, a reconciliation, or a slow moving ahead. We run the risk of being bored with solutions.

WHEN WE focus on the solutions and don't get our identity from the problems, we may discover that our lives are a lot healthier even if a bit less "exciting."

❧ June 10

PERFECT CONTENTMENT

Perfect contentment can rarely be recognized. Maybe in Tibet—maybe in toddlers.

—Carrie Fisher

Perfect contentment may be one of the most important states that we will ever have the opportunity to recognize in ourselves in our entire lives. It's probably there—just buried a bit under the surface—and I have no doubt that it's there.

Of course we're busy. Of course we do too much. Of course we're under pressure. Of course we're tired. Of course we're overwhelmed at times. So what?!

Down deep we like our work, now don't we? We love all the benefits we get from it.

We love our children. They are so funny and cute and we never know what they are going to say or do.

We even can love our tiredness. We are tired because we have been doing a good job and that feels good.

We can even take some pleasure in feeling overwhelmed. We wouldn't have so much to do unless we were good, and we can do it, now can't we?

Contentment is an active place of quietude, a busy place of stillness. We remember it—even if vaguely.

SO-O-O-O, ALL we have left to do is dig under all that other stuff and find that place of perfect contentment that is there in each of us because of who we are and what we are doing. We're good!

❧ June 11

BEAUTY

Adornment is never anything except a reflection of the heart.

—Coco Chanel

Everyone pays so much attention to how women dress: "We should wear three-piece suits, look just like men, and dress for success." "Women who get raped were asking for it by the way they dressed." "Men like women who dress in a feminine fashion. It makes men feel masculine."

Is it any wonder that we sometimes feel confused about what seems right for us to wear?

What if the way we dress is simply a reflection of our hearts? What if our main criterion for beauty is what feels good on our bodies and reflects who we are? What if we wear colors because we like them and not because they are "our colors" or make us look thin? This opens up all kinds of possibilities, doesn't it?

IF I ADORNED MYSELF **to reflect my heart, what would I wear?**

❧ June 12

JUST BEING

> *I never lose sight of the fact that just being is fun.*
> —Katharine Hepburn

No matter how busy we are, how much we have to do, how many demands are made on us, we can still be having fun.

Demands, deadlines, and schedules can never keep us from "just being" unless we let them. Just being doesn't take a lot of time. Just being can occur while you are busy with the tasks of life.

Just being can happen while you are watching TV, cleaning up the kitchen, changing the sheets, changing a diaper, or making a knockout presentation.

Just being is not relegated to those stolen moments of a soaking bath, yoga, or meditation. Just being can be sneaked into any little crevice that is our life—and it's so much fun.

JUST LIKE WE don't have to wait for the "big discovery" to do something great, we don't have to wait for that special moment to just be and enjoy it completely.

✢ June 13

LIVING LIFE FULLY/CURIOSITY

Life was meant to be lived and curiosity must be kept alive. One must never, for whatever reason, turn his [sic] back on life.

—Eleanor Roosevelt

As I look back over the significant teachers in my life, one of the characteristics that consistently stands out is their curiosity. We sometimes think that curiosity is reserved for youth and is only natural in young children.

Yet I am sure that if we think about the people we have known, those that we remember most vividly are those who remained incurably curious throughout their lives.

There is an intimate link between curiosity and aliveness. Curiosity appears to be in the gene bank of the human species. My curiosity is not dead, even though it may seem to have been slumbering for a while.

MAY I NEVER BE **"cured" of my curiosity!**

⁂ June 14

AWARENESS OF PROCESS/WISDOM

The events in our lives happen in a sequence in time, but in their significance to ourselves, they find their own order . . . the continuous thread of revelation.

—Eudora Welty

Wouldn't it be boring if our lives were completely linear? How dull to have completely worked through each experience and trauma right when it happened!

Yet we all become resentful when old skeletons that we believed were long since buried begin to rattle their bones. How inconvenient when the effects of events that happened at age five begin to erupt at age thirty-five! How disquieting when memories long hidden from consciousness signal us that they are ready to be worked through!

Can we believe that our own inner process knows when we are ready to deal with old issues? Can we trust that the very fact that they are coming up is an indication of how much we have grown and how strong we are?

THERE IS SOMETHING **within me that knows more than I know. Trusting it can only result in healing.**

❧ June 15

CONFUSION/NEGATIVISM

Why is it when I don't know what I want, there is always someone waiting to tell me what it is? I'm just lucky, I guess.

—Anne Wilson Schaef

I have heard so many women say, "I have a good marriage. My husband doesn't beat me, he doesn't gamble, and he doesn't run around with other women." Or they say, "Well, my job isn't boring, it keeps me busy, and it pays the bills." Somehow, OK becomes the absence of awful. If something in our lives isn't too destructive, it must be all right.

We get so confused about what we really want and what is really good for us. We are so accustomed to doing what is expected of us that we have lost our ability to determine what we want.

UNLESS I KNOW what I want and what is right for me, there is no way I can be an honest person.

✤ June 16

BEING CRAZY

> *What sane person could live in this world and not be crazy?*
>
> —Ursula K. Le Guin

How easily we believe that *we* are the crazy ones! Maybe this just isn't true, Maybe we need to take another look at who's defining crazy.

Given, we overdo, run around like crazy, try to take care of anyone in sight (during a deposition once I began to feel so sorry for the opposing lawyer who was taking my deposition that I was tempted to "help her out." My lawyer called a recess and said, "What are you doing?" "I feel sorry for her. She's going to hang herself," I said. "Let her," he snapped back. Sigh!), and, in general, buy into the insanity.

Do we need to buy in? Do we want to buy in? Just because the world around us is crazy, we don't have to be.

Have you listened to the news lately? It's the "no spin" people who have the greatest "spin." Why wouldn't we feel crazy? We have spent years trying to fit into crazy situations and be successful there.

MAYBE it's time for us to give up trying to be as crazy as our surroundings and be the clear, sane women we are.

❧ June 17

SHARING FEELINGS

> *For the most part fear is nothing but an illusion. When you share it with someone else, it tends to disappear.*
> —Marilyn C. Barrick

Those ideas that we hold in our heads and in our bodies can become so toxic that they begin to feed on themselves. In our busyness, we can store them away to dwell on and have little or no awareness that we are doing it. They become illusions that are running our lives.

For example, I have long known the magic of talking. When I am angry about something, the minute I say I am angry, almost magically, the feelings go away and I am faced with a different reality. And then, of course, I have to deal with a new reality.

When I am afraid and I say I am afraid, I shift to another reality. It's not that I wasn't really afraid. I was. And, when I give the feeling words, the fear changes. This shift is one of the magical processes about speaking our feelings. No one knows why the shift occurs, and it does. We can secrete our feelings and cause them to fester and grow or we can share them with someone we trust.

TALKING is good. Sharing our fears is good. And be prepared for a shift.

❧ June 18

LIVING IN THE PRESENT

I know the solution. When we have a world of only now with no shadows of yesterdays or clouds of tomorrow, then saying what we can do will work.

—Goldie Ivener

Imagine starting each day fresh with no "shadows of yesterdays or clouds of tomorrow." In our more negative, cynical moods, we hear such an idea and we scoff, impossible! It is not possible to let go of the past and have no concern for the future. Yet this is what every great spiritual teacher on this planet has taught in one way or another. In fact, the greatest gift our spiritual teachers have given us has often been to show us how to live in the present, how to simply be totally present to the moment.

How often we miss our life by focusing on the past or yearning for the future. We miss the look in our children's eyes today, because we are thinking about how to get them to the dentist tomorrow. We miss the interesting idea that has just now come across our desk, because we are worrying about what we said in the meeting yesterday. Stop—relax—be here!

THE PRESENT is all I have: to leave it is to kill it.

❧ June 19

ACCEPTANCE OF SELF

> *Do nothing because it is righteous or praiseworthy or*
> *noble to do so; do nothing because it seems good to do so;*
> *do only that which you must do and which you cannot*
> *do in any other way.*
>
> —Ursula K. Le Guin

We are so accustomed to doing what others want us to do, or doing what is right, or doing that which earns us praise, that LeGuin's words urging us to do only that which we *must* do and cannot do in any other way seem unrealistic. We think: That's fine for her to say, she's a writer—she schedules her own time.

Yet, what truth is there for us in her words? We certainly can admit that we have done many things for the wrong reasons, and the pain of our righteousness, "nobility," or praise-seeking is often bitter in our hearts. Often when we do something because it seems good to do so, we waste everyone's time, including our own.

What a relief to believe that we are enough just as we are and that our unique way of accomplishing a task is just what is needed.

I WILL sit with these ideas. After all, who else could make my contribution!

✖ June 20

EXPECTATIONS

Life's under no obligation to give us what we expect.
—Margaret Mitchell

Expectations are real killers! They are setups for disappointment. Often, because of our expectations, we are completely oblivious to what is really going on in a situation. Because we are so wedded to what we think *should* be happening, or what we want to happen, we don't see what is happening.

Many a possible relationship has been aborted because we were too determined to turn it into *a relationship*.

Expectations also keep us in illusion. We set up our expectations for someone, we project them onto the other person, and then we start reacting to our expectations as if they were real. Expectations and the illusion of control are intimately linked.

When we are tied to our expectations, we usually miss what's happening . . . life, that is.

EXPECTATIONS **are premeditated resentments.**

❧ June 21

MY LIFE

My life is not up for criticism, just my work.

—Cher

For women who do too much, this is a tough one. Can we separate our life from our work? Is work more our life than our life? If we are raising children, have we made them our work and we don't have a life other than as their mother (a burden for them!)?

No matter what it is that we do, do we have a life, our life?

Each of us was given a life. That life is ours. Do we know how to live it?

We may share our life with our husbands, lovers, friends, family, and colleagues, and we don't do well when we ask them to define our lives for us.

We are always comparing ourselves to others: no matter what we have or who we are, it never quite seems to be enough. We are always too much or too little, too fat or too skinny, too intelligent or not intelligent enough, too assertive or not assertive enough. In comparison, we always lose.

When we go to work, to our children, to our relationships, we need to bring someone we know intimately—ourselves. And, that someone is best received when we have something of unique interest, intellect, creativity, or wisdom to share.

WHEN WE have a life, we can then say, "My life is not up for criticism, just my work."

❧ June 22

THE EBB AND FLOW

> *Life comes in clusters, clusters of solitude, then clusters*
> *when there is hardly time to breathe.*
>
> —May Sarton

We workaholics, busyaholics, and rushaholics feel much more familiar with and comfortable with times when we hardly have time to breathe. We know how to function under pressure and with deadlines hovering over us. These times are when we shine.

Unfortunately, it is the time of calm and potential solitude after the project is finished that scares us. To be without a project or a deadline strikes terror in our bones. Fortunately, we rarely have to deal with that terror because we have arranged our lives in such a way as to rarely have a "breather."

If we take time to notice, this ebb and flow in life has a reason. We need breathers. Our bodies need to rest from our constant adrenaline push, or they blow up.

As we let ourselves get healthier, we begin to experience and treasure the "clusters" of our lives and welcome them as examples of infinite wisdom.

THE OCEAN never tires of the ebb and flow of the tides. I have something to learn from the ocean.

❧ June 23

THANK YOU

And who knows? Somewhere out there in this audience may even be someone who will one day follow in my footsteps, and preside over the White House as the president's spouse. I wish him well.

—Barbara Bush

Well, whadda ya know? The wife of George and the mother of George W. is a closet feminist. Even Nancy Reagan said, "Feminism is the ability to choose what you want to do. I'm choosing what I want to do."

It's interesting how certain terms go out of style in our culture—feminism, addictions, liberalism—yet the concepts and the social ills behind them still stubbornly persist. In fact, they may persist even more strongly without the consciousness of the label. Instead of looking down our noses at the women who bore the labels, we might want to take a minute and thank them for the work they did for us so that we have the possibility to be president and see if women can make a change or to make choices for our lives, our children, our creativity, and our strong beliefs. As Sandra Day O'Connor says, "Young women today often have very little appreciation for the real battles that took place to get women where they are today in this country."

IT NEVER HURTS to say "thank you" to those who have given us presents.

❧ June 24

COURAGE

This is the art of courage: to see things as they are and still believe that the victory lies not with those who avoid the bad, but those who taste, in living awareness, every drop of the good.

—Victoria Lincoln

How aptly put! Courage is not just seeing things as they are, which is vastly important; courage is accepting reality with the ingenuity to continue to see and experience the many good things that happen to us.

I remember in graduate school I acquired the nickname "Pollyanna," because I always could see something interesting and exciting in everything that happened. I did not always like those grueling reports and seemingly sadistic examinations and yet, when I was honest with myself, I always had to admit that I had learned something when I finished. Because of the nickname and the subtle judgmentalism attached to it, I began to question myself. After some reflection, I realized that a pollyanna was someone who denied the negative and only saw the positive. I did not do that. I saw and accepted the negative and delighted in whatever positive there was. As a consequence, graduate school was not difficult for me. Working has not been hard for me either.

A SMILE, a nod in the elevator, a few minutes of quiet time—these are living every drop of the good.

❧ June 25

BEING POWERFUL

Our deepest fear is not that we are inadequate. Our deepest fear is that we are powerful beyond measure. It is our Light, not our Darkness, that most frightens us. We ask ourselves, who am I to be brilliant, gorgeous, talented, fabulous? Actually, who are you not to be? You are a child of God. Your playing small does not serve the world.

—Marianne Williamson

These words resonate. Even Nelson Mandela has used them in one of his speeches. Why are we so afraid? It is as if our fear of inadequacy is blown up to cover up our deep knowledge that we are "powerful beyond measure."

Why wouldn't we be afraid? We have seen those who stick their neck up above the crowd get their head chopped off. Okay. So there's a risk. We've dealt with risks before, haven't we? Of course we have.

Do we need to be afraid of our light, being gorgeous, talented, brilliant, and fabulous? Do we owe it to our Creator to be as filled with light as possible and as powerful as we can be?

MAYBE one of the reasons we do too much is so we won't have to deal with the light that is within us and truly know how powerful we are.

❧ June 26

LIVING LIFE FULLY

When I speak of the erotic, then I speak of it as an assertion of the life force of women; of that creative energy empowered, the knowledge and use of which we are now reclaiming in our language, our history, our dancing, our loving, our work, our lives.

—Audre Lorde

What a wonderful opportunity today is to celebrate ourselves as women! To celebrate ourselves does not mean that we put men down or do not like men. We are only celebrating ourselves and the unique contribution that women have made, are making, and can make.

All of us have gifts that are unique to us. No one else has quite the combination of gifts that each of us has to offer and many of those gifts are not in spite of being a woman, they are *because* we are women. Not to share the fullness of our woman gifts is a form of stinginess, and no one likes to be stingy.

MY EROTIC **is my life force. I can have fun with this.**

❧ June 27

ACTION

If you want a thing well done, get a couple of old broads to do it.

—Bette Davis

If there is anything we "old broads" know how to do, it is to get things done. We women are so practical. We have an uncanny ability to see what needs to be done, roll up our sleeves, and do it. We are rarely too proud, too prissy, or too elitist to do what needs to be done. We thrive on the ordinary.

Sometimes we fail to see how important our practical everydayness is. We long for the great inspiration, the important recognition, or the big breakthrough. Yet all our lives are made up of common tasks that need to be done. When something is common and ordinary, we frequently fail to see its real importance. What we do is important, and we do it well. Failing to see that is a form of dishonesty. And we don't want to be dishonest, do we?

I AM a competent "old broad." Maybe I can appreciate myself for the way I consistently tackle the everyday.

WHOLENESS

Don't you realize that the sea is the home of water? All water is off on a journey unless it's in the sea, and it's homesick, and bound to make its way home someday.
　　　　　　　　　　　　—Zora Neale Hurston

We are all like water. We are off on a journey to return to ourselves. Some of our journeys have taken us far afield, and many of our days have been absorbed by the sandy riverbanks that contain us. Yet we continue to flow—heavy and swollen in the spring of our lives and often reduced to a trickle as we approach the fall of our years. "Return, return, return," we murmur, as we tumble over the stones in our paths, ever cognizant that although we may wander through new and strange lands, our destination is a return.

WATER has to return to the sea, just as I have to return to me.

❧ June 29

SELF-AFFIRMATION/POWER

> *Think of yourself as an incandescent power, illuminated*
> *perhaps and forever talked to by God and his [sic] mes-*
> *sengers.*

—Brenda Ueland

As we begin to get more in touch with ourselves and accept ourselves for who we are, we begin to entertain the thought that we might, indeed, be "an incandescent power." We begin to feel our power and know it not as power over others, but as personal power, glowing within.

As we clear out the garbage of our crazy behavior, we uncover a spiritual being lying dormant, not dead, within us. We have a sense of what it means to be in tune with the infinite, and life feels easy and flowing. This feeling of oneness is not an illusion; it is real. Only as we learn to affirm who we are do we move beyond ourselves.

AS WE AFFIRM who we are, we become even more of who we are.

🌿 June 30

JOY AND HAPPINESS

> *Joy is what happens to us when we allow ourselves to recognize how good things really are.*
>
> —Marianne Williamson

Yeah! Right! How good things really are. I have a phrase I utter that has become very important to me. It is "I'm quite happy."

This phrase has a life of its own in my life. I can be driving down the road and suddenly I will burst out, "I'm quite happy." I can be sitting watching one of my favorite programs on TV accompanied by the purrs of my big white cat and suddenly "I'm quite happy" rolls out of my mouth. Or, I can be working at my desk, getting something done that needs to be done and feeling quite pleased with the outcome and "I'm quite happy" trips gaily through my brain.

A strange phenomenon occurs at these times. I have discovered that when the words actually form, I am even happier.

JUST ADMITTING joy and happiness seems to engender more.

❧ July 1

NICENESS

I haven't been being nice . . . I've been chicken.
                                        —Claudia

As women we have been trained to be nice. We *do* "nice" things for people, we *say* "nice" things, and we *are* "nice." Many of us fear that if we stop being nice, we have to become nasty. Having become bored with our niceness, many of us have experimented with nasty.

For those of us trying to get clearer with ourselves and others, we have discovered that our niceness is intimately linked with our dishonesty. If we want to be more honest, we have to be willing to let go of our "niceness." In letting go of our niceness, we find ourselves becoming more honest. Getting honest about ourselves and our lives is an essential step toward health. To be more honest, we also have to give up being chicken and put ourselves out there.

OFTEN, **when we say we are being nice to protect other people, the person we are really protecting is ourselves.**

❧ July 2

LIVING LIFE FULLY

I have made a great discovery.
    What I love belongs to me. Not the
    chairs and
tables in my house, but the masterpieces of the
world.
    It is only a question of loving them enough.
                    —Elizabeth Asquith Bibesco

We get so embroiled with possessions. We find ourselves feeling that we need to own places, persons, and things. We try to possess our lives, and we believe that we can. We need to learn from the butterfly that alights on our hand. If we watch it and admire it, as it chooses to stay for a while, we are blessed with its beauty. If we try to hold on to it, we will kill it. It is in the not trying to possess that we have.

Imagine what it really means that we can have all the treasures of the world—not to own, but to appreciate, to enjoy . . . to live with.

AM I CAPABLE of loving so much that I am able to appreciate that which I do not possess? I hope so.

✺ July 3

HUMOR

> *Yo' ole black hide don't look lak nothin' tuh me, but uh*
> *passel uh wrinkled up rubber, wid yo' big ole yeahs flap-*
> *pin' on each side lak uh paih uh buzzard wings.*
>
> —Zora Neale Hurston

I love the writing of Zora Neale Hurston. She has a way of cutting right through to the meat of things, and she does it with humor and clarity. How often have we had thoughts similar to those quoted above, and we haven't let ourselves enjoy the tickle and the giggle in our own minds? We make life so *serious* and everything so important that we don't dare laugh—it might offend. We might offend.

In order not to offend, we render ourselves and our lives humorless. How dull.

I THINK it might be helpful to remember that our humor adds color to a world gone grey with inattention.

❧ July 4

UNDERSTANDING

The most sympathetic of men never fully comprehend women's concrete situation.

—Simone de Beauvoir

And, when we get right down to it, most of our situations are concrete. It's not that we don't understand "abstract." We can handle abstract just as well as men and do. Yet, we women are often left with the concrete of day-to-day living—the wife business, the maid business, the mother business, the detail business. These are the places where men don't "comprehend."

The reality is that we understand men and their way of doing things just fine. We don't always agree (often) and we don't always like it (not much), and we understand it. We have to in order to live in this culture. Men don't have to understand us or the way we do things to live in this culture. That's the truth of it. They have to try (maybe) to be in relationships with us and not for their survival.

We women have spent eons trying to make ourselves understood by those who can't possibly understand us.

The failure isn't ours. Let it go. We both get battered in the process.

WE ALL **need women friends, regardless of how good our relationships with the men in our lives are.**

❧ July 5

PRISONS

I create my own prisons. No one else is putting these walls around me.

—Michelle

Rarely do we recognize the construction of our enclosures until they are already built. We are fooled by their illusionary appearance: they look like security, prestige, power, influence, money, and acceptance. It is only when the construction is completed that we realize that we are enclosed in splendid isolation. When did it happen? We looked down at our work or our lives for only a second, and then looked up to find that our illusions of security have become a benevolent prison. Prisons have room for fantasies, but prisons have little room for dreams.

We have misjudged our priorities. We do not want the isolation of success at any cost. Somehow, we thought we could "have it all" and now all of it has us.

MY ISOLATION has been of my making, so my reaching out for help can also be of my doing.

❧ July 6

FORGIVENESS/AMENDS

Her breasts and arms ached with the beauty of her own
forgiveness.

—Meridel LeSueur

To ache with my own forgiveness is to be wholly accepting of myself. None of us is without need of forgiveness. We have all done injury to those closest to us. This is one of the most painful aspects of our lives: we hurt those we love the most. We hurt ourselves when we hurt those we love. When we are preparing to make amends to others, we must first make amends to ourselves and forgive ourselves for the wrongs we have done. Only then can we be truly ready to make our amends to others.

There is, indeed, a beauty in our forgiveness of ourselves. We can be simple, direct, and without fanfare in our forgiveness of ourselves.

I AM in need of forgiveness. I am in need of forgiveness of myself.

❧ July 7

FRIENDS

From the first time I met the little girl until her death recently, a period of a little over seventy years, we were friends.

—Mrs. Mary E. Ackley

"We were friends"—such a simple yet powerful statement: "We were friends." How many of us can truly say that we are a friend?

One of the devastating realities of busyness and doing too much is that we progressively have less and less time for friends.

We have to make appointments for friendship. Hanging out with a friend seems a luxury or even an inconvenience. Or we assume that we are friends and never do anything to nurture the relationship. We treat our friends like we treat ourselves, and that's not very nice.

IT IS NOT POSSIBLE to live a rich, full life without friends. I have to be one to have one.

❧ July 8

GROWTH

My favorite thing is to go where I've never been.

—Diane Arbus

To go where we have never been, whether internally or externally, is always exciting. This excitement may be covered over by fear and trepidation. Yet I have always found that somewhere deep inside of us we are excited when we have the opportunity to explore the unknown.

Men are not the only explorers. We women are explorers too. Our explorations may take different forms: we love to try out a new recipe; we love to try out a new idea or ideology; we love to visit new places and learn from different cultures. We are especially adept at courageously launching into hidden and unknown areas in ourselves and others. In spite of our fears, there is a deep quest for our truth in each of us.

I PREFER a road map on my journeys, and I am willing to go without one if I must.

❧ July 9

ENTHUSIASM

> *One needs something to believe in, something for which one can have whole-hearted enthusiasm. One needs to feel that one's life has meaning, that one is needed in this world.*

> —Hannah Senesh

Several years ago, I made a drastic decision for myself. I decided that I would do only work that I was enthusiastic about. I was a psychotherapist, speaker, and workshop leader then. This decision was very frightening for me, since I was a single parent and had many financial responsibilities.

I decided not to accept any clients about whom I wasn't enthusiastic. I would not do any speeches or workshops just because of the money, or prestige, or ego. I would do only what seemed *right* for me to do. I would do only things that intuitively seemed related to the meaning and purpose of my life. I feared I would end up a derelict, a bag lady, and starve, yet, I have had more money since that decision than I ever had before. I still live my life based on that decision.

I'M NOT SAYING this will work for everybody, *and* it worked for me.

❧ July 10

ADMITTING OUR REALITY

I'm anal retentive. I'm workaholic. I have insomnia. And I'm a control freak. That's why I'm not married. Who could stand me?

—Madonna

Well, she is married now, at least. And doesn't she sound just like the successful woman of today, which she is?

Is this what we women who do too much are striving for— success accompanied by obsessive behavior, workaholism, insomnia, and being a "control freak"?

This description doesn't look that good when we see it on paper, does it?

Let's be a little forgiving of ourselves here. This busy syndrome is not exactly how we planned our lives, is it? I doubt it.

If we really stopped to take an honest look at our lives, we would probably have to say that the present situation crept up on us when we were blindsided. We can't really believe this is what we had in mind. Can we?

The good thing Madonna does is admit and accept her reality as it is now.

IF WE admit and accept our reality as it is now, we have the opportunity to change it—if we want to, that is. Honesty is always good for us. Especially honesty with ourselves.

❧ July 11

WHAT'S NEXT?

The only thing that makes life possible is permanent, intolerant uncertainty: not knowing what comes next.

—Ursula K. Le Guin

How can she say that? Where on earth is she coming from? What can she possibly mean? Isn't it just like a writer to say something like that so we have to ponder what she means? We don't have time for this kind of nonsense.

Well, maybe we better take the time, because understanding what she means may shift our worlds.

We have spent so much time and energy trying to order our worlds, make things permanent, eliminate uncertainty. Don't we have schedules, appointments, marriages, weatherproof houses, and insurance policies for everything just to take care of this mess?

Please, please don't tell us we're on the wrong track.

Just ask yourself one question. If you could have had complete control of your life and could have made it static to stay just the way you wanted it at each "perfect point," would you have had as much fun and learned as much as you have? We just don't have that much wisdom, imagination, and creativity.

WE REALLY **don't know what's coming next anyway, do we?**

❧ July 12

GUILT/ALONE TIME

I wanted to drive up here alone and several people asked if they could drive up here with me. I can't tell you how hard it was just to come by myself.

—Mary

Often we feel guilty when we do something for ourselves. We have so accepted the mandate to be aware of others' feelings, take care of them, and put ourselves last that we often feel uncomfortable if we even *have* needs. How selfish it seems to refuse a ride to someone who needs it when we are going that way anyway. Surely we could put ourselves out a little. Even if we do refuse the request and get our time alone, are we going to be so overcome with guilt that we won't enjoy the time anyway? What a lose-lose situation!

Maybe we can use that time alone to explore our gift of guilt and learn from it. Even having time to explore our guilt requires alone time. We may need that exploration desperately.

WHEN I SAY no to a request for my time, I am not going away from that person, I am going to myself.

BEING IN CHARGE

I'm not going to limit myself just because people won't accept the fact that I can do something else.

—Dolly Parton

There is a vast difference between trying to control our lives and taking charge of our lives. Trying to control our lives puts us in a position of failure before we start and causes endless, unnecessary pain and suffering.

Taking charge of our lives means owning our lives and having a respond-ability to our lives and then letting it go. Taking charge of our lives means that we do not spin our wheels with impression-management and try to be. It also means that we do not accept their evaluation of what we cannot be and stop there.

WHEN I LET GO of my need to control, I am in a better position to be in charge and to receive information from my power greater than myself.

❧ July 14

BEING TORN

At work, you think of the children you have left at home. At home, you think of the work you've left unfinished. Such a struggle is unleashed within yourself. Your heart is rent.

—Golda Meir

Being torn seems to be an accepted given for women who run a home and also have other work. Many of us have tried to be superwomen and have almost pulled it off. Yet even when it appears that we are "making it" and successful in both arenas, we are aware that internally we feel torn and guilty in relation to our family. Frequently, this results in our taking our frustration out on our children, which results in more guilt. We feel like a violin string pulled taut and about to break.

Perhaps it is time to sit down with our families and tell them how we feel. They probably need to hear that we really *want* to be with them and that we do not know how to balance our lives. They may even feel relieved to know that our lives feel overwhelming (which everyone but us has admitted!).

JUST PLAIN HONESTY **works for so many things. Perhaps I really shouldn't just save it for special occasions.**

QUESTIONS

I'm tired of being labeled anti-American because I ask questions.

—Susan Sarandon

When did asking questions become a negative?!

As children, we had a million questions, and even though some of the adults in our lives became exhausted by them, questions were seen as positives. We were viewed as having inquiring minds and that was good.

As we grew older, we still had a lot of questions—sex (a lot about sex, as I remember)—trying to understand and explore our world and learn how to be an adult in it.

Then, we became an adult and questions suddenly became off-limits. We were expected to know everything and be expert at everything. We were expected to know how to raise children, how to run a household, how to run an office, how to compete and win in the fast-paced world in which we live.

No one had time or energy for our questions, and we didn't have time and energy to ask them. Questions had become unpopular and annoying and bothersome.

WHAT IS LIFE **if it does not include asking questions and seeking answers?**

❧ July 16

BALANCE

Creative minds have always been known to survive any kind of bad training.

—Anna Freud

Even though her father believed that our lives are determined in our first five years, Anna Freud seems to have moved beyond him. Although we are affected by our past and our training, each of us has within us the possibility to move beyond both.

Unfortunately, when we try *not* to be like our parents, we get caught in the same trap as when we feel that we *have* to be like them. Either way we are determined by our past and controlled by our reaction to our past. Some of us spend our entire lives vacillating between these two positions.

We do have another choice. That choice is to acknowledge our past and be ourselves.

THE THIRD option is to be me. That is where my creativity lies.

❧ July 17

DOORS

I have become my own version of an optimist. If I can't make it through one door, I'll go through another door—or I'll make a door. Something terrific will come no matter how dark the present.

—Joan Rivers

When we are speeding around like those automobile ads on TV, so busy that we dare not look up, we don't have much time for seeing doors. Even if we catch a glimpse of a possible door, we are well past it by the time our mind registers that may have been a door.

Could it be that our life is more difficult than it needs to be because we are unable to see the doors of opportunity that are presented to us every day? Could it be that we have fallen prey to the habit of constant rushing to such an extent that we don't know how to slow down? Could it be that we are actually afraid of slowing down? Are we afraid that if we slowed down and actually saw one of those doors and went through it that we would have even more work and not less?

We could miss an opportunity to do something we had wanted to do for a long time. We might not notice the opportunity to do something nice for someone. We could miss that essential piece of information that would make all the pieces fall together

CAN WE trust that if we slow down enough to see and explore the doors of our lives that "something terrific will come"?

❧ July 18

DOING THE BEST WE CAN

I feel that God gives us these children and expects us to do the best we can with them for a certain time. Then they are on their own.

—Betty Ford

Every parent does the best she can. We may think that ours have done a pretty horrible job—or, at least, it seems like that until we have children of our own. Then, we begin to see that even *our* parents did the best they could given the parenting they had and the life circumstances they encountered.

I don't want to shock you, and, in all fairness, I feel this needs to be said. NONE OF US HAD PERFECT PARENTS AND NONE OF US WILL BE PERFECT PARENTS.

Being a parent is anything but easy, and, paradoxically, sometimes the best thing we do is simultaneously the worst we do. We look for directions and no one has a road map for parenting. We want to work so our own children will have more advantages and yet it means we have less time with them. Nothing is easy. Little is clear.

There. With that said, maybe we can settle down to just doing the best we can with everything we do even if we have no children. Then, we can let go after that.

WHEN WE **get right down to it, if we do the best we can that's enough, and it's really all we can do.**

ALONE TIME/BEING RESPONSIBLE

For every five well-adjusted and smoothly functioning Americans, there are two who never had the chance to discover themselves. It may well be because they have never been alone with themselves.

—Marya Mannes

Superwomen can always be heard to say, "I know that having time to oneself is important. It's just not possible for me. I just have too many responsibilities."

One always wonders how women who seem so powerful and so much on top of their lives can become so helpless in determining what they do with their time. Our helplessness seems to be situational and often emerges only in relation to *our* needs.

As successful women, we are often least successful in caring for ourselves. We need skill training in self-help.

THE CHOICES I make about what I do with my time are *my* choices (even when they don't appear to be!).

❧ July 20

NEGLECT

> *Show me someone who never gossips, and I'll show you*
> *someone who isn't interested in people.*
>
> —Barbara Walters

Have we been neglecting our family and friends by not gossiping about them? Do we even have time for a good gossip session with "the girls" anymore?

While we're at it, have we been neglecting a lot of things lately? What about calling our parents and friends? What about a relaxed lunch with someone we dearly love who we haven't seen for a while?

What about our children? Are we doing the "right" things with them, like activities, practice sessions, and homework, and not really spending relaxed, unpressured time with them?

Do we have to make an appointment to spend time with our spouses?

And what about ourselves? When was our last medical exam, teeth cleaning, pap smear, facial, or massage?

IT'S VERY IMPORTANT **to notice what and who we have been neglecting and do something about it.**

❧ July 21

AVOIDING CRUTCHES

> *Now some people when they sit down to write and nothing special comes, no good ideas, are so frightened that they drink a lot of strong coffee to hurry them up, or smoke packages of cigarettes, or take drugs or get drunk. They do not know that ideas come slowly, and that the more clear, tranquil and unstimulated you are, the slower the ideas come, but the better they are.*
>
> —Brenda Ueland

One of the side effects of our doing too much is that we begin to use chemicals and other addictive substances to keep us going. Then our addiction to doing too much becomes compounded with a complex array of other addictions.

Another side effect of being women who do too much is that we find ourselves progressively out of touch with our creativity and our productivity.

Brenda Ueland uses the focus of becoming a writer to call us back to ourselves. Yet, the truth in what she is saying applies not only to writers, it applies to all of us. Our creativity and productivity always suffer when we use addictive substances to try to force them.

I DON'T NEED to *do* something for my creativity to emerge. I probably need to *stop* doing some things.

❧ July 22

SUCCESS

Life is a succession of moments. To live each one is to succeed.

—Corita Kent

Perhaps it is not the concept of success that is the problem, it is the way we define success. If we define success as lots of money, getting to the top of the organizational ladder, two BMWs in our garage, and a designer house, success may be dangerous to our health.

If we define success as living each successive moment to its fullest, we may have money, prestige, and possessions, and this success may *not* be disastrous to our health. The difference is in the attitude and in the beliefs behind that attitude.

In fact, it is often easier to gather the accoutrements of success than it is to live a successful life. Living a successful life demands our presence, our presence in each moment.

SUCCESS gets confusing. Is it what I have or what has me? Probably neither.

❧ July 23

CONFIDENCE/CYCLES

> *Everyone has bad stretches and real successes. Either way, you have to be careful not to lose your confidence or get too confident.*
>
> —Nancy Kerrigan

It's probably just as debilitating to believe that the successes will go on forever as it is to believe that the bad stretches will never end. They are both really similar, you know. Each is a phase. Each is a process. The difference is how we treat them.

With the successes, we try to hold on to them. We clutch them close and say, "Please, please, please stay." We become overconfident.

With the bad stretches, we fight them with every ounce of our being, try to ignore them, and beg them to go away. We lose our confidence when we cannot make them go away.

How much energy we spend and waste trying to make our life look like we think it should. No wonder we are exhausted!

At a very deep level, our life has its own process. It is made up of cycles, and the sooner we attune to these cycles the sooner we will have energy for other things.

IF I tie my confidence to the cycles of my life, my confidence will be on a roller coaster.

ACCEPTANCE/HUMILITY

> *But if you go and ask the sea itself, what does it say?*
> *Grumble, grumble, swish, swish. It is too busy being the*
> *sea to say anything about itself.*
>
> —Ursula K. Le Guin

No one who has ever sat beside the sea and experienced her eternal power and gentleness can have any question that the sea knows that she is just that, the sea. Nature has such an ability to be exactly what she is, with no pretense . . . and she does not even have to stop and think about it.

When we have to stop and think who we are, we are not being who we are. When we are trying to be someone we believe we should be, we are not being who we are. When we are trying to be what someone else has told us we should be, we are not being ourselves. To be myself, I have to *be*.

NATURE **teaches great lessons in humility. In order to learn from her, I have to be in her.**

WONDER

> *I take a sun bath and listen to the hours, formulating, and disintegrating under the pines, and smell the resiny hardihood of the high noon hours. The world is lost in a blue haze of distances, and the immediate sleeps in a thin and finite sun.*

> —Zelda Fitzgerald

I read the above passage, and I feel lost in wonder— wonder at the beauty of the words and phrases. I read it and I remember the wonder of a spontaneous sunbath in a light-speckled woods where the sun on my skin enhanced the mixed scent of forest musk and pungent pine, as the smells permeated my body. I can remember listening to the hours as they initially crashed around me, then gradually smoothed into a murmur as my body relaxed into the earth and into myself. The world seemed far away, and there was no need to bring it closer.

WONDER is a gift of living. Living is a gift of wonder.

❧ July 26

TRUST

> *Nature has created us with the capacity to know God, to experience God.*
>
> —Alice Walker

We often think that we have to work to know God and that we have to have experts to teach us how to know our Higher Power.

What a wonderful surprise it is suddenly to discover that the capacity to know God and be connected with our Higher Power dwells within us and to discover that instead of working at this connection, we have only to admit that it is already there. We may have lost our awareness of our relationship with our Higher Power, and the connection has never stopped. It is only that our awareness of it has dimmed and become obscure.

I HAVE all I need within me to know and experience my Higher Power. All I have to do is step out of my way.

🌿 July 27

PERFECTIONISM/LONELINESS

> *"She happens to belong to a type [of American woman]
> I frequently met . . . it goes to lectures. And entertains
> afterwards . . . , amazing, their energy," he went on.
> "They're perfectly capable of having three or four chil-
> dren, running a house, keeping abreast of art, literature
> and music—superficially of course, but good Lord, that's
> something—and holding down a job into the bargain.
> Some of them get through two or three husbands as well,
> just to avoid stagnation."*

—Dodie Smith

It sort of grates to see ourselves described on paper.
We have learned to cope. We have learned to be superwomen. So what if we don't go very deeply into anything. How can we? We just don't have the time. Our
biggest fear is not knowing enough or not being enough.
We feel that we are inadequate if we cannot talk intelli-
gently about almost everything and do almost anything.
We would like to have more intimate relationships, but
we just do not have the time—we are perfect women.

WE ARE **perfect women, and being perfect is boring to
ourselves and others.**

TOXIC PEOPLE

Toxic people. Research has shown that the emotional pain they create in your life is associated with tension, sickness, physical breakdown, and disease.

—Christiane Northrup

One of the characteristics of people who live in a dysfunctional situation is that we develop an increased tolerance for insanity.

We have seen this phenomenon in the battered women syndrome. On the outside, people can easily see what is going on and say, "Why does she stay?"

Inside the situation, our perceptions are quite different. After a while of being around toxic people, we stop noticing the battering, the meanness, the put-downs, and the rejections. So much of our energy is taken up with survival that we have none left for noticing.

We need to step back and notice the toxic people in our lives. We can get support to do just that.

ONCE WE notice that we have toxic people in our lives, we have a myriad of options for healing and taking care of ourselves.

❧ July 29

HAVING A LITTLE FUN

> *If it is true that men are better than women because they are stronger, why aren't our sumo wrestlers in the government?*

—Kishida Toshiko

When I read the above quote, I had the most wonderful image. When someone is making a complete fool of himself in government—or anyplace else for that matter—what would happen if a sumo wrestler just sat on him? It's an intriguing possibility and a great image.

One of the wonderful aspects about our minds that we probably don't use nearly enough is the pleasure we can get from the images that pop into them.

These kinds of images are perfect for women who do too much. They're easy—we don't have to do much at all—in fact, our minds do it for us.

They're instant. They flash in and out in a second—no time required—no waiting here.

They're pleasurable—a bit of fun with no time, money, or energy expended.

And . . . *our mental images work.* We always feel better.

ONE TIME when I was going into a meeting I anticipated would probably be difficult and even hostile, I had a flash of myself sitting in red cowboy boots and a tattooed Maori warrior standing behind me with scowling face, war club, and crossed arms. I giggled throughout the meeting (and bought the boots later!).

❧ July 30

CONTRADICTIONS

If I could see what's going on with myself as well as I see what's going on with others, I'd be "fixed" by now.

—Pat

So much of our lives are glaring contradictions. We swear that we will never be like our mothers, then find ourselves screeching on the same note. We know we would never manipulate others the way our boss manipulates us, and then we catch ourselves doing it.

We seem to see so clearly "out there," while "in here" is a muddle. Relax, it's all part of denial. Breaking through the denial about what is really going on in our lives is the first step to healing.

MAYBE what we notice "out there" is what we need to see "in here." I'll check that out.

HAPPINESS/DEPRESSION

When a small child . . . I thought that success spelled happiness. I was wrong, happiness is like a butterfly which appears and delights us for one brief moment, but soon flits away.

—Anna Pavlova

There is no difference between happiness and depression. They both have the same process. It is just the content that is not the same. Both will come and go. The major difference between them is what we *do* with them.

We are always seeking happiness. When we see it coming we say, "Ah, come here, I see you. Stay with me always." Happiness laughs and says, "Oh, she's seen me, I can leave now." And it does.

With depression, we see it coming, and we say, "Go away, I don't want you. Not me." And depression sighs and says, "Here we go again, I'm going to have to get bigger and bigger for her to hear me and learn what I have to teach." So it taps us on the shoulder and says, "Over here, over here!" until it gets our attention. Then it leaves.

Both happiness and depression have something to teach us. Both will come and go. Both will return. It is our response and openness to learn from both that makes the difference.

MY HAPPINESS is a gift. My depression is a gift. Both are like butterflies in my life.

❧ August 1

JOYFULNESS

Not all songs are religious, but there is scarcely a task, light or grave, scarcely an event, great or small, but it has its fitting song.

—Natalie Curtis

How long has it been since we let ourselves savor the pure joy of listening to music? I am not talking about the songs on the radio that we crowd in as we speed along the freeway. I am talking about the sheer joy of bathing ourselves in the music we like the most.

Likewise, how long has it been since we have let ourselves hear the song of the task we are doing? When we do too much, we lose our joy in the doing and see only the labor and the deadlines. Even when we do not see the song in our work, it is still there. We have but to listen.

TODAY **I have the opportunity to open myself joyfully to the music around me.**

❧ August 2

HOLIDAYS/VACATIONS

Travel not only stirs the blood . . . It also gives strength to the spirit.

—Florence Prag Kahn

Part of the destructiveness of being women who do too much is that we don't take the time for those things that "stir the blood" and "give strength to the spirit." We simply do not take time for vacations and trips with those we love. And even when we do, we frequently do them like we do the rest of our life—rushing, pressured, and frantic.

Vacations mean a change of pace, a gentleness with ourselves, a time of rest and renewal, and a time to stretch ourselves and encounter new people, new lands, new ways, and new options. The very newness opens the possibility of expanding our spirits and flushing out the stagnant particles in our blood.

WE OWE it to ourselves and those around us to take vacations.

❧ August 3

FREEDOM

> *Would you sell the colors of your sunset and the*
> *   fragrance*
> *Of your flowers, and the passionate wonder of your*
> *   forest*
> *For a creed that will not let you dance?*
>
> —Helene Johnson

Would you? Have you? What kind of creed have we accepted that tells us that we are of no value unless we are working ourselves to death? What kind of creed have we adhered to that tells us that *doing* is superior to *being*? What belief have we accepted that suggests that, if we are not rushing and hurrying, we have no meaning?

We don't have time for sunsets, fragrances of flowers, or the "passionate wonder of our forests." We don't even see sunsets, flowers, or forests. Do they still exist?

Dancing surely must be for pagans who don't have to make money. We used to dance before we became so important.

WHEN a creed is not articulated as a creed and is assumed to be reality, we don't have much freedom of choice.

WORK/TRUTH

> *I was brought up to believe that the only thing worth doing was to add to the sum of accurate information in the world.*
>
> —Margaret Mead

We live in a time of intense information exchange so rapid that it boggles the mind. We are constantly bombarded with news items, new scientific information, new ideas, and new possibilities. Where do we fit? What is our place in all this?

As women, we often discount our knowledge and try to skew our information or our perceptions so that they are acceptable to others. In so doing, we rob the world of our accumulated knowledge. Accurate information is important to the world. Accurate information from a variety of perspectives is *essential*.

I DO have a place and my information is important.

❧ August 5

HARMONY AND COMMON DESTINIES

> *A spirit of harmony can only survive if each of us remembers, when bitterness and self-interest seem to prevail, that we share a common destiny.*
>
> —Barbara Jordan

A spirit of harmony—sounds peaceful and comforting, doesn't it? In our homes . . . at our work . . . in our churches . . . in our volunteer organizations . . . a spirit of harmony.

Bitterness and self-interest have become so integral to the warp and woof of our commercial, materialistic, high-pressured, money-centered society that it is more and more difficult even to remember harmony and sharing a common goal.

Could it be that the high pressure and the constant busyness of rushing around obliterates our memory of harmony and a shared destiny?

Yet this country was founded on both harmony and shared destiny—a diverse mob of people striving toward the same goals.

Maybe we have put too much emphasis on the striving and not enough on a common destiny and harmony.

WE HAVE to slow down a bit to remember what is important to us. We feel better and have more energy when we remember what is important to us.

❧ August 6

GRATITUDE

> *Big Blue Mountain Spirit,*
> *The home made of blue clouds . . .*
> *I am grateful for that mode of goodness there.*
>
> —Apache chant

It is impossible to come into contact with Native American spirituality and not be struck with the immensity of the gratitude expressed. Theirs is a gentle, quiet, flowing form of gratitude that runs as deep as the still lakes and soars as high as the peaked mountains. The Native American form of gratitude is peaceful. This peacefulness permeates all their legends and stories.

Sometimes we feel that if everything isn't perfect, we cannot be grateful for anything. We easily fall into all-or-nothing thinking. When we do, we miss the sunrise and the other forms of goodness that surround us.

I AM GRATEFUL. **Perhaps that is enough. I am grateful.**

❧August 7

GROWTH

Character building begins in our infancy and continues until death.

—Eleanor Roosevelt

Somehow, we always have the secret hope that we can get ourselves together, work out all our issues, discover all our talents, accept our life's work, and then relax and get on with it.

What a shock it is when we finally recognize that "character building" and growth are lifelong processes and continue throughout our lives. Just when we think we are clear about the direction of our lives, and we settle into that security (stagnation), something shakes our complacency. How much easier it is to recognize in the first place that life is a process and to open ourselves to the cycles of growth in ourselves.

TO GROW and develop is the normal state for the human organism. . . . I am a human organism. It would be logical, therefore, to assume that growth and development are normal for me.

❧ August 8

EVERYDAY GENIUS

My routines come out of total unhappiness. My audiences are my group therapy.

—Joan Rivers

We spend so much time and energy waiting for the right time, wishing for the right circumstance or hoping for the big break. We are often so busy with the rush of hoping, wishing, and anticipation that we miss what we have to work with here and now.

Geniuses are not necessarily people who have all their ducks in order and everything laid out for them as they would like them. Geniuses are people who take what life presents to them and make something innovative and clever out of it. Geniuses are women who look at an almost empty cupboard and fridge and come up with a gourmet meal. Geniuses are everyday women who shift their perspective ever-so-slightly and create newness.

Joan Rivers turns unhappiness into a lucrative comedy routine.

IT'S NOT ALWAYS **what we were dealt; it's how we use it that works or doesn't.**

❧ August 9

LIVING MY LIFE

Dying is a wild night and a new road.
—Emily Dickinson

Emily Dickinson was present to the process of her dying when she said these words. She seemed to be fully with herself and, at the same time, open to what would come. When we think of our own death, most of us hope that we can be open to the moment.

All too often, the idea of dying and the experience of slowly killing ourselves through overwork is something with which we have become comfortable. It is the living of our lives at each moment that terrifies us and that we seek to avoid.

Luckily, we can get through this terror and come to know that we have all the caring support we need to live our lives.

THIS IS MY MOMENT. I will live each moment. Then death will be a culmination, not an end.

❧ August 10

GOALS

To have realized your dream makes you feel lost.
                                    —Oriana Fallaci

Several years ago one of my friends called me in a panic. "Anne," she said, "You have to do something immediately! There are some women really hurting out there and nobody knows!"

She had been interviewing women who had been in top executive positions for seven to ten years. She said it was as if they had made the team, and every day they got suited up, got on the bus, and went to the game, but . . . they never got off the bench. At first they were hopeful, but after a few years they had become resigned to the reality that they would never quite belong.

She said that she found more alcoholism, clinical depression, and anorexia-bulimia in this group of women than she had ever seen.

IT IS NOT **the realization of our dreams that makes us feel lost. It is what happens to us when our dreams become nightmares.**

❧ August 11

BUSYNESS

We are always doing something . . . talking, reading, listening to the radio, planning what next. The mind is kept naggingly busy on some easy, unimportant, external thing all day.

—Brenda Ueland

What lengths we go to keep away from ourselves! We have such an inability to relax. There are always just a few more tasks we can get done. Sometimes it almost seems that we are afraid of what might happen if we let our minds be idle for even a moment. We fill in every crack and crevice with activity. Sometimes, we even try to crowd two or more activities in at once, like making out a list of things that need to be done while we watch the news, or directing the activities of the kids while we are working on a report.

We have become habituated to busyness, and if we are not busy we feel worthless, at a loss, and even frightened.

NOTICING **how busy I keep myself is the first step. Realizing that I am powerless over this busyness is the second. Recognizing that my busyness is adversely affecting my life is next.**

❧ August 12

INTIMACY

With my workaholism, my intimacy skills deteriorate to almost nothing.

—Emily

Whoops! We have developed new skills. We know how to be efficient. We know how to be productive. We know how to be organized. We can give orders with the best of them. We're better at math and numbers than anyone ever believed possible. We're respected. We're admired—maybe even feared.

Just because we have developed new skills doesn't mean that we have to let the old ones deteriorate or be let go completely.

We women are the intimacy experts. The world of intimacy, as with Atlas, rests on our shoulders. We know how important intimacy is. We believe in intimacy. We want to be intimate with ourselves, intimate with those we love and intimate with life. How can we let our intimacy skills deteriorate when we so believe in intimacy?

WE *are* intimacy . . . lest we forget.

❧ August 13

A MAN'S WORLD

*The art of being a woman can never consist of being a
bad imitation of a man.*

—Olga Knopf

Our mothers fretted about our fathers being type A
personalities and dying young. They enjoyed the
advantages that their spouses working long, hard
hours provided. And they complained about lack of
companionship, raising the children alone, and meals
grown cold because of "getting tied up at the office."
They saw their husbands working themselves to death,
felt helpless, and feared really having to raise their
children by themselves. They worried about those
women at the office who were more interesting, and
feared affairs that would make their husbands feel
more alive.

But things have changed. We are modern women. We
don't have to fuss and complain about our absent husbands working themselves to death. We are doing it ourselves. We don't have to worry about our husbands
having affairs—neither of us has the energy for affairs.
Affairs take time and energy.

We have developed the same high blood pressure,
high cholesterol, heart disease, diabetes, and stroke-
prone lives as our husbands. We've made it. We have it all.

NOW THAT WE have it all, we may want to take a very
close look at what we have lost.

EXPECTATION/SUCCESS

> *My expectations—which I extended whenever I came close to accomplishing my goals—made it impossible ever to feel satisfied with my success.*
>
> —Ellen Sue Stern

A lot is never enough for women who do too much. Whenever it looks like we may have the experience of successfully completing a project, we add on other contingencies and set up the possibility of doing even more than we originally had thought possible.

Sometimes we even make tasks more complicated than they need be so we can keep busy. We feel safer when we are working. We get panicked with slack time. We feel it is almost impossible to let ourselves savor our successes. And, if we would be truthful, we have many of them.

IT'S ALL RIGHT to have successes. It's even all right to be successful.

❧ August 15

BUSYNESS

I'm a workaholic. If I'm not working I exercise. If I'm not exercising, I eat. I don't ever stop from morning to night.
—Terry

Some of us have modeled our lives after the roadrunner cartoon character: jump out of bed—beep, beep. Throw in a load of laundry so it can wash while we do our exercises and shower—beep, beep. Nine minutes for make-up and hair—beep, beep. Seven minutes for starting the coffee, getting dressed, and popping in the toast. Five minutes for eating breakfast and making out a list of things that must be done today—beep, beep. Throw laundry into the dryer, grab coat, purse, and briefcase, and burst through the front door—beep, beep.

By the time we have finished our morning routine, most people would be exhausted, and we have just begun—beeep . . . beeep. . . .

PERHAPS it is important to remember that I was not created to be a roadrunner, even if we have some features in common.

✳ August 16

> *However, one cannot put a quart in a pint cup.*
> —Charlotte Perkins Gilman

There is a Zen story about a college professor who came to a Zen master seeking knowledge. The old Zen master looked over the professor carefully and then asked a student to go fetch her a pot of tea and two cups. She then placed a cup in front of the professor and began to pour. The tea filled the cup and spilled out over the table. Seeing this, the professor shouted, "Stop, can't you see the cup is full? It can hold no more!" The old Zen master smiled and said, "And so it is with you. Your mind, too, is full of too many things. Only when you empty it will there be room for more knowledge to come in."

Asking for help is a way of "emptying" our lives. Stopping and seeing that our lives have become too full may well be the beginning of a process that can empty us and make way for new ways of being.

MY CUP runneth over may in some contexts be a declaration of disaster. Emptying is fully as important as filling.

AWE

> *But what will never, never change is the wonder, the*
> *indescribable wonder to me of seeing Earth lying in*
> *space as in the hollow of God's hand.*
>
> —Zenna Henderson

Awe is a feeling that is rare in our busy lives. Awe means stopping and noticing. Awe is, at least momentarily, letting ourselves remember and experience the vastness of the universe or the amazingly intricate design in the petal of a tiny flower.

One of my friends from Germany came bearing gifts when she visited. The most intriguing was a tiny one-inch-square magnifying glass which unfolded such that the distance between the end of the stand and the magnifying glass was a little over an inch, exactly the distance needed to see clearly the tiniest veins in a leaf, the detail on the back of a bug, or the center of a minute flower. This little device opened up an entire universe to my awareness. What she had really given me was a gift of awe.

LIFE **without awe is like food without herbs or spices.**

❧ August 18

INNER KNOWINGS

Yes, my voices were of God. My voices have not deceived me.

—Joan of Arc

Sometimes we try to ignore our "voices." We even try to convince ourselves they are "insanity."

Yet we all have "voices"—intuition, "knowings," dreams, sudden awarenesses. Sometimes it feels as if we women carry the burden of these subtle knowings for the entire culture, since we live in a time of "proving it," substantiating our findings, providing the scientific proof.

Yet, we "know" and we know we know. We don't always know *how* we know and we know. Asking us to "un-know" is like asking us to cut off a limb. And, the abuse we get for these "whisperings," these "knowings," is mighty. As Lily Tomlin says, "Why is it when we talk to God, we're said to be praying—but when God talks to us, we're schizophrenic?"

TRUSTING **our inner knowings is a tough one.**

❧ August 19

YOUTH

> *Youth is, after all, just a moment, but it is the moment,*
> *the spark that you always carry in your heart.*
>
> —Raisa Gorbachev

How lucky for each of us that we have had our youth. Of course, there is more and more pressure to "be" our youth no matter how old we get. Ignore that.

Let's remember our youth. One of the powerful dangers of doing too much is that we have little or no time for nostalgia and remembering. That's too bad! For nostalgia and memories are two of the sweetest gifts we have as human beings.

Regardless of what went on in our youth, we had a youth. We had the bubbliness of youth. We had the moments of sweetness of youth. We had the curiosity of youth. We had the discovery of youth. These promises come with being young, not just looking young, and they are ours to treasure throughout our lives.

A MOMENT for remembering, for nostalgia, and for letting yourself feel the spark of youth is so refreshing to the soul.

❧ August 20

SADNESS/MOVING ON

If ever I had a good mind, it has been lost in the shuffle. I seem to have stagnated, and I am aware that I am not using any capacity I have to the fullest.

—Anonymous

Resignation . . . despair . . . a sadness in lost possibilities. It's time to take stock and realign our priorities. We seem to have wandered off our path. Perhaps we have even forgotten what our path was.

Maybe it is time to feel the grief of lost opportunities and stagnating minds. Life often teaches us through our wrong turns and missed possibilities. This feeling of sadness may well be the door to a new beginning. But we will never go through the new door if we do not let ourselves go through the grief and sadness.

As we let ourselves feel our grief and pain, we will truly have the opportunity to step onto a new path and to explore our lives.

MY GRIEF and pain are mine. I have earned them. They are part of me. Only in feeling them do I open myself to the lessons they can teach.

DUTY

Duty should be a by-product.

—Brenda Ueland

Duty can be a tyrant that we can pull out to justify inhuman behavior toward ourselves and others, a hard taskmaster that suffers no leeway, a monster that we carry on our head and shoulders.

There's nothing wrong with duty. We just should not let duty override our clear feelings and intuitions. Duty cannot come before our own internal clarity. When it does, it is a tyrant. Duty needs to follow our clarity, just as doing things for our loved ones needs to be an expression of love, rather than ritualized behavior. Duty needs to be a by-product of who we truly are, and what we value, and what is important to us.

RITUALIZED **duty is a sham!**

✣ August 22

WONDER

> *If a child is to keep alive his inborn sense of wonder without any such gift from the fairies, he needs the companionship of at least one adult who can share it, rediscovering with him the joy, excitement, and mystery of the world we live in.*

—Rachel Carson

How fortunate if we get to be that adult who has the opportunity to be a companion to a child and support that child's sense of wonder! We are lucky because that child can offer us the opportunity to rekindle our own awareness that wonder continues to dwell in us. That child can remind us that we still have the capacity to look at cloud formations with new eyes and to giggle in excitement with a new discovery. How long has it been since we really had a belly laugh, especially at ourselves? How long has it been since we saw a rainbow in a drop of rain? How long since we studied the progress of a red and black ladybug on our hand?

I WONDER where our wonder is?

STRUGGLE

> *You wear yourself out in the pursuit of wealth or love or*
> *freedom, you do everything to gain some right, and once*
> *it's gained, you take no pleasure in it.*
>
> —Oriana Fallaci

Sometimes we forget what's important. We struggle so long to establish ourselves that we become addicted to the struggle. We begin to think that if we are not struggling we are not alive. In fact, the excitement and intensity of the struggle become our complete focus, so that we forget our original goal.

There is no doubt that we as women have had to struggle individually and as a group. Yet, if we become like those against whom we struggle, we may find that we have lost ourselves in the process.

SOMETIMES we have to struggle . . . sometimes not. The issue is not the romance of the struggle; the issue is who we are as we engage in it.

❧ August 24

SECRETS

As awareness increases, the need for personal secrecy almost proportionately decreases.

—Charlotte Painter

As Isak Dinesen says, "a secret is an ugly thing." We are as sick as the secrets we keep.

Often we fail to recognize the effect that secrets have on our lives. They are like a quiet cancer that eats away at our souls and devours our relationships. When we enter into a contract of secrecy with someone, we give a little piece of ourselves away. If we give away too many pieces of ourselves, we are devoured, very much like the heroine in Margaret Atwood's novel *The Edible Woman*.

An important part of recovering our souls is to give up secret-keeping. It is only when we live our life in the open, accept responsibility for the decisions that we have made, and own our behavior that we begin to know health.

AS THE FRENCH say, "Nothing is so burdensome as a secret."

HAPPINESS/CONTROL

They seemed to come suddenly upon happiness as if they had surprised a butterfly in the winter woods.
—Edith Wharton

Happiness, like most of the other important processes of life, cannot be planned. We often come to believe that if we just had an important job, plenty of money, the right relationship, attractive and intelligent kids, and a lovely home, we would be happy. When we attain these goals and still secretly feel depressed, or not quite fulfilled, we immediately ask ourselves, "What's wrong with me?"

We have done all the things that are supposed to bring us happiness, and we don't feel any better. Where have we gone wrong? We always question ourselves and believe that there is something innately wrong with us. It takes us a long time to stop and question the system that taught us that accumulation and control are the vehicles to happiness.

HAPPINESS is a gift. We cannot make it happen. It comes like "a butterfly in the winter woods." Let it sit with us a while.

❧ August 26

RAISING CHILDREN

If you bungle raising your children, I don't think whatever else you do matters very much.

—Jacqueline Kennedy Onassis

Sometimes it's just too overwhelming to let ourselves know what a big responsibility we have taken on by choosing to have children.

We loved the idea. Our hormones and our fantasies pushed us. We wanted to have it all. And now, well, to realize the magnitude of this decision seems a bit much.

There are some very important things to remember about raising children.

First of all, most mothers feel overwhelmed. That's just the name of the game. We are not alone.

Second, children are not a task to be completed, a meal to finish, or a report to submit. They're much more complex. Children are a process—a process of living. Our best choice would be to participate in that process as much as possible. Forget goals, participate. Also, we worry about the responsibility to teach them what they need to know and forget that it is equally important to let them teach us, even if we are slow learners—remembering that maybe our child chose us because we had so much to learn.

Also, remember that children are very resilient and forgiving or no one would have ever grown up. Of course we'll bungle sometimes.

WORRYING about bungling raising our children may be our biggest bungle.

❧ August 27

LONELINESS

Because they are cut off from their internal power source, they really feel alone and lost.

—Shakti Gawain

When we think about what is missing from our lives, we may come to the conclusion that *we are!* Oh, of course, we function well. We do the things that need to get done. We are even efficient and imaginative at times, and yet so often we feel like zombies carrying out an old routine in well-worn ruts. We have lost touch with ourselves, and there is nothing lonelier than not being in touch with ourselves.

When we have lost ourselves, no amount of externals will help. Spouses, friends, work—none can supply what is missing when we are cut off from our "internal power source." *We* are missing, and the only way to remedy this problem is to find ourselves again. Finding ourselves takes time. It is hard work *and* it is worth doing.

I WAS **looking all over for what was missing in my life, and then I discovered** *I* **was.**

❧ August 28

CELEBRATIONS

The more you praise and celebrate your life, the more there is in life to celebrate.

—Oprah Winfrey

Aren't celebrations great?! I celebrated my fiftieth birthday for two years. I started the day after my forty-ninth and ended the day before my fifty-first. During that time, I decided to let myself do some of the things I had been putting off, and really wanted to do.

A week ago, I celebrated the life of one of my dear, dear friends. He died a week before his ninety-second birthday and had gathered much wisdom during those years.

The day after, I celebrated being with friends and having some time to write.

Two days later, I celebrated a day with some newly met Australian Elder friends and had dinner with some dearly loved longtime friends.

The next day, I celebrated by going to the Korean Spa and having a complete facial and Korean massage.

The next day, I celebrated by going by a friend's gallery and having an "art feast" seeing her new shipment of tapestries.

And the next day, I went to a movie and potluck to celebrate a wonderful trip and the completion of the *Women Who Do Too Much Calendar* for next year.

ISN'T THIS **how life is supposed to be? Everything can be a celebration. Celebrations are not just for special occasions.**

IMPRESSION MANAGEMENT

Women's virtue is man's greatest invention.
—Cornelia Otis Skinner

How much we distort ourselves in trying to please others. Women have historically been controlled by the demands and expectations of others. We have been so willing to let others define us and so eager to fit that definition that we have lost all track of who we are.

As we come more in contact with ourselves, we realize that many of the definitions of who women "naturally are" are generated to take care of others. For example, it has been an accepted truth of psychology that women are "natural nesters," and men the "wanderers." Yet, in recent times, when women have been getting divorced, it appears that it is the men who quickly find another woman to make a nest for them, while women become the wanderers. So many of our definitions of who we are have been invented for us by others, to please them and meet their needs—and we have desperately tried to fit their images of what is acceptable.

A VIRTUOUS **woman is someone who is herself.**

INTRODUCTION

INTERRUPTIONS

> *It is distraction, not meditation, that becomes habitual;*
> *interruption, not continuity; spasmodic, not constant*
> *toil.*

—Tillie Olsen

How we hate interruptions, especially when we are working on something important. In fact, when we are working on something important, everything is an interruption. As Tillie Olsen says, distraction, interruption, and the spasmodic seem to be our lot sometimes.

How difficult it is to mesh the process of our life and the process of our work. Yet, how sweet it is when that happens!

One of the reasons that "meditation," "continuity," and "constant toil" have not been possible is because we have not believed that we deserve the time for ourselves to do our own work. Just as the addict who is into her self-centeredness is out of touch with herself, the workaholic who is into her workaholism is out of touch with her work.

WHEN I TRUST my process, I trust the process of my work.

❧ August 31

ALONE TIME

> *So you see, imagination needs moodling,—long, ineffi-*
> *cient, happy idling, dawdling and puttering.*
>
> —Brenda Ueland

What wonderful words: moodling, dawdling, and puttering! I have a friend who says that she likes to "frither." The word sounds just like what it is: putzing—really doing nothing.

I used to have a big dog named Bubber who was one of my most important teachers. He used to sit out on our deck up in the mountains and just look. It was difficult for me to imagine what he was looking at all the time, so one day I just went out and sat beside him and "looked." I sat with him for a long time and experienced just sitting and just looking. I learned to take time just to sit and look. One sees so much when one just sits and *looks*. Doing nothing else . . . just looking.

Bubber has since died, and his great wisdom in having taught me to sit and look lives on.

NOT ALL of us can have Bubbers, *and* all of us can frither and putz.

✽ September 1

HONESTY

I give myself sometimes admirable advice, but I am incapable of taking it.

—Mary Wortley Montagu

How refreshing when we can be honest, even humorously honest, about ourselves! Often we are so busy protecting ourselves that we don't dare risk letting others know that we aren't perfect. Of course usually we are the only ones fooled by our masquerades, but we make ourselves believe that others are fooled, too.

When we can be honest with ourselves, we usually know very clearly what we need and what is destructive to us. The trick is, can we listen to ourselves? Are we capable of following our own good advice? Can we let ourselves see our foibles and laugh about them? After all, no one knows us as well as we know ourselves. So, naturally, we are the persons who are most capable of seeing ourselves clearly. Are we courageous enough to let ourselves see ourselves and be honest about what we see?

ADVICE is difficult, even when it comes from ourselves. Even if we can't put our advice into action, we don't need to beat ourselves up about it.

❧ September 2

JOYFULNESS/CONTROL

In search of my mother's garden I found my own.
—Alice Walker

One of the greatest joys in life is to be in search of one thing and to discover another.

Before we became more aware, we were so controlling that surprises struck terror in our heart even when they were wonderful. We just didn't want anything coming at us that wasn't planned, structured, and under control. We now realize that trying to control everything has been one of the ways that we have robbed ourselves of the joy of living.

No wonder life has seemed dull at times—we have made it that way. It's not that the potential for joy wasn't there. We just were too busy and controlling to notice it.

THE PURE joyfulness of the unexpected can be a source of wonder to me.

❧ September 3

IN TOUCH WITH A POWER
GREATER THAN ONESELF

Those who lose dreaming are lost.
—Australian Aboriginal proverb

If we are to have any hope of being in touch with the process of the universe or with a power greater than ourselves, we must learn to move beyond our rational, logical minds and to let ourselves "dream."

That does not mean that there is anything wrong with our rational, logical minds, but we can have trouble connecting with a force greater than ourselves when we *lead* with our rational minds.

The ancient Huna teachings tell us that we consist of three parts: a conscious self that runs our day-to-day living, a higher self where we are one with the Creator, and a lower self that is feelings, memory, intuition, dreams, and more, and that our conscious self can only access our higher self through our lower self. Interesting!

There are so many things in this universe that affect us and with which we are connected. Sometimes the only way we can be aware of that connection is to let ourselves dream beyond our knowing. We have so much to learn from everything around us, if we just open ourselves to that which may be.

I ADMIT **I don't know it all yet. Learning comes in many forms.**

❧ September 4

LEARNING

Patterns of the past echo in the present and resound through the future.

—Dhyani Ywahoo

We are a process, and the key to living that process is learning. Mistakes are not proof that we are bad; they are doors for learning and moving on. If we have no memory, we can't learn from our past. If we have no past, we have no present and we have no future.

Everything in our lives is an opportunity for learning. Often, our most painful experiences open doors that must be opened before we can take our next steps. That doesn't mean that we don't sometimes have to walk over what seem like beds of hot coals to reach the door. Yet once we reach the other side the learning is there.

Kurt Vonnegut talks about "wrang-wrangs" in our lives, great teachers who are placed in our path. The lessons they teach us are vastly important, and they are taught through struggle, pain, trial, and tribulation. Still, they are important teachers.

THE NEXT TIME a "wrang-wrang" drops into my life, I have the option to recognize that person as a teacher.

❧ September 5

Discoveries have reverberations. A new idea about oneself or some aspect of one's relations to others unsettles all one's other ideas, even the superficially related ones. No matter how slightly, it shifts one's entire orientation. And somewhere along the line of consequences, it changes one's behavior.

—Patricia McLaughlin

How amazing we human beings are! One little change in any aspect of our life affects so many other facets of our being in as yet unimagined or undreamed of ways that we never really quite know where anything will lead. We say no to something at work that for many months we have wanted to say no to and instead of the backlash we expected, we experience some subtle indication of respect. We certainly respect ourselves more.

We break our necks to earn respect and admiration, only to discover that we really have no control over how others perceive us. Our letting go of our illusion of control in even the smallest way reverberates throughout our lives.

I KNOW that gradually, ever so gradually, I am growing and changing. My life is much more like a mobile than a ladder. Each new discovery affects every aspect of my being.

❧ September 6

RECOGNITION/SELF-ACCEPTANCE

It's amazing how much people can get done if they do not worry about who gets credit.

—Sandra Swinney

This is a tough one for us women. We have spent so many years seeing others get credit for what we have done. We have fought like tigers to be recognized and have our contributions recognized and appreciated.

Now, how can we move on? Proving ourselves isn't what we want either.

We'll never have acceptance unless we first give it to ourselves. Once we truly accept ourselves and our contributions, maybe outside recognition may not be so important. And, it certainly is nice, though.

To ride the tide of self-acceptance is to rise above the need for recognition. Getting credit may not be as important as getting what we want done.

PERHAPS WE CAN start with looking at ways we do not feel accepting of ourselves.

✤ September 7

DEMANDING TOO MUCH OF ONESELF

I believe that IQ's change, and mine dropped considerably. I'm no longer very competent in any area. My children all turned out well not due to me, but rather to a strict father who allowed no nonsense.

—Anonymous

What has happened to this woman? Where did she go? As we read what she says about herself, we have the feeling that she is disappearing before our very eyes. Many of us have had the experience of being devoured by our families, our houses, our jobs, and our lives. I once knew a woman who used to keep looking back for footprints on the sidewalk, because she had the strange feeling that her soul was seeping out through the soles of her feet.

I can remember feeling as if I did not exist as a separate person when I used to work at the kitchen counter and my children would stand on my feet to make themselves just a little higher. Or, when they wanted to get from one end of the couch to the other and they just walked over me as if I were not there. Life can, at times, invite us to disappear.

Yet, how arrogant it is for the woman quoted above to accept that her children turned out well and to believe that she had nothing to do with it! What a dedication to self-abnegation!

TODAY, I WILL be willing to look at the possibility that my self-battering is an arrogant and self-centered activity that is not useful to me or anyone else.

❧ September 8

AMBITION

Sometimes you wonder how you got on this mountain.
But sometimes you wonder, "How will I get off?"

— Joan Manley

Ambition has been important to many of us. When we were little girls, we realized that it was important that we work hard and become somebody. We wanted to get ahead, and we were willing to go to any lengths to be competent and important. In the past few years women have had many more options for our lives, and we wanted to take advantage of these opportunities.

When did things change? When did we cross over the line from having ambition, which was good, to being had by our ambition, which is killing us?

Often, the very skills that kept us alive when we were younger (like dishonesty, control, and manipulation) are now lethal and are draining the life from us. This may be true about our ambition. If it now is running our lives, it may be time to take another look.

WHAT WAS GOOD for us at one stage of our lives may be lethal now. We need to take stock and see where we are with our lives.

❧ September 9

WISDOM

> *Women have always been the guardians of wisdom and humanity which makes them natural, but usually secret, rulers. The time has come for them to rule openly, but together with and not against men.*
>
> —Charlotte Wolf

It is time to listen—to listen to myself and to listen to the ancient wisdom that is all around me.

Women are such masters of practical wisdom and we live in a world that is dying for lack of practicality. What good is the best invention in the world if it doesn't *work*? What good are the best ideas in the world if we cannot use them?

If we are indeed the guardians of wisdom, it behooves us to share that wisdom.

AS MERIDEL LESUEUR SAYS, **"The rites of ancient ripening / Make my flesh plume."**

❧ September 10

STARTING OVER

The two important things I did learn were that you are as powerful and strong as you allow yourself to be, and that the most difficult part of any endeavor is taking the first step, making the first decision.

—Robyn Davidson

These words were written by a woman who learned to handle camels and traveled alone with them across the Australian Outback. Somehow the intensity of the circumstances under which she gathered these learnings makes them even more profound. What if each of us believed that we are "as powerful and strong" as we allow ourselves to be? What if we quit trying to be accepted by everyone and gave up trying *not* to alienate anyone and just let ourselves be as strong and powerful as we are? Nothing extraordinary, mind you, just as wonderfully powerful as we naturally are.

And, what if we let ourself take that first step toward what we really want? Nothing big . . . no fanfares . . . just do it!

DO I HAVE **any idea how powerful I can really be?**

❧ September 11

SERENITY

> *The silence of a shut park does not sound like country silence; it is tense and confined.*
>
> —Elizabeth Bowen

When we are not really dealing with our doing too much, we are often silent and not serene. We have only shut up for a while and are still "tense and confined," like a city park shut off from activity.

Serenity is more like having a "country silence" within. Serenity is an acceptance of who we are and a *being* of who we are. Serenity is an awareness of our place in the universe and a oneness with all things.

Serenity is active. It is a gentle and firm participation with trust. Serenity is the relaxation of our cells into who we are and a quiet celebration of that relaxation.

LONGINGLY, way back somewhere, I remember what it is like to have a "country silence" within. I can be grateful for that sense of knowing.

❧ September 12

REACHING OUR LIMITS

I have had enough.

—Golda Meir

What beautiful words, and how rarely are they spoken by women who do too much. Part of our craziness is not recognizing that we have limits and then not knowing when we reach them. In fact, many of us may see having limits as an indicator of inadequacy. We cannot forgive ourselves for not being able to carry on when we are exhausted or for not being able to keep going regardless of the circumstances.

Recognizing that we are approaching our limits and accepting those limits may be the beginning of wisdom.

EVERY **human being has limits, and I am a human being.**

LIVING LIFE FULLY

> *She wants to live for once. But doesn't know quite what that means. Wonders if she has ever done it. If she ever will.*
>
> —Alice Walker

Most of us would like to live life fully. Yet when it comes to putting those words into practice, we are not quite sure how. We wonder if we know what living life fully really means, or if we have ever known.

Our temptation is to rush out and stock up on "how to" books. If we can just find the right book, we will know what to do. We have read enough so that we are pretty good at following directions. Or we start going to lectures and workshops. We try meditation, drumming, chanting, special diets, special exercises, and special therapies. Always looking outside ourselves for the formula and answers.

At some point we realize that in spite of how good all these approaches are, we have to come back to the realization that only *we* know how to live *our lives* fully. We can accept guideposts, and ultimately, living our lives is up to us.

EVEN IF we have never done it, the knowledge of how to live our lives fully lies deep within us.

❧ September 14

FEELING OVERWHELMED

Feeling overwhelmed isn't surprising. Being surprised about it is.

—Anne Wilson Schaef

Is it any wonder we often feel overwhelmed? Just the bills for all the "necessities" of life seem more than we can handle sometimes. And then there are federal income taxes, state taxes, changing deductions, investments, sales, best buys, 10,000-mile checkups on our cars, teeth cleaning, pap smears, travel arrangements, and planning family vacations, if we dare to take one.

Recent estimates on the rate of information processing tell us that every few minutes we process more information than was processed in a lifetime by those living in the Middle Ages.

Feeling overwhelmed feels like a normal reaction.

SOMETIMES **it helps to know that I just can't do it all. One step at a time is all that's possible—even when those steps are taken on the run.**

❧ September 15

FEELINGS

Sorrow is tranquility remembered in emotion.

—Dorothy Parker

How lovely! All feelings are equally as lovely.

We have done ourselves such a disservice by talking about "negative" and "positive" feelings. Feelings are just feelings, and like every other aspect of our being are gifts from which we can learn.

Sorrow and grieving are feelings that we try to avoid. They take time and are not easy. Yet we make them worse by avoiding them. We feel sad when some promotion doesn't come through. We feel sorrow when we lose those we love. How beautiful to think of it as "tranquility remembered in emotion."

Grief is real, and it is human. We grieve our losses, whatever they are. Grief is an unfolding process that has many levels. It is important for us to accept our passage through the levels of grief. It is even normal to feel grief when we finish an interesting project, or when our company or family restructures.

IT IS FIGHTING **our feelings that causes our suffering, not our feelings.**

❧ September 16

VAGUE STRUCTURE

If I stick to this vaguely, I will get more accomplished.
—Jacqueline Kennedy Onassis

I love it! The above was written on the edge of her schedule. What a role model! Make a schedule—schedule appointments if you will—stick to it vaguely, and you'll get more accomplished.

Real productivity and certainly creativity never come from sticking to something slavishly. Life is just not that neat and clean, and when we try to make it that way we are the ones who suffer, along with what we are trying to accomplish.

Some things don't take as long as we thought they would. Others take longer. The time in between the scheduled tasks may be the most important time of all. Only by hindsight can we realize what was most important.

PERHAPS IT'S our vaguely structured flexibility that will serve us best in the end.

GIFTS/WORRYING

> *I think these difficult times have helped me to under-*
> *stand better than before how infinitely rich and beauti-*
> *ful life is in every way and that so many things that one*
> *goes around worrying about are of no importance what-*
> *soever.*

> —Isak Dinesen

It's not that we need to seek pain and suffering to glean the rich learnings of life. When they happen, how-ever, we learn so much more if we can see these situations as rich opportunities for learning. We spend so much time worrying, and worrying is nothing more than an attempt at remote control. Often what we worry about never comes to pass. Unfortunately, we may be so preoccupied with worry that we miss the gifts our life is presenting to us at the moment.

When will we realize that the unfolding process of our lives is so much richer and varied than we ever could have planned? The unplanned and uncontrollable gifts we receive add color to the tapestry of living.

I NEVER KNOW in advance what will be an important gift for me. Hence it behooves me to be open to possibilities and not ever waste time worrying.

GUILT

I even feel guilty about feeling guilty.

—Nicole

Women are the first in line to stand up for a good cause. We can mobilize an army of volunteers to save a faltering school system, a crumbling church, or a sagging corporation. We are willing and able to put our weight behind any cause that is politically correct. We genuinely care about the homeless, the starving, the brutalized, and the forgotten, and we do a great deal of good. Who knows how much of our causes are motivated by guilt? Only we can know that, as we look inside.

The one cause that we have difficulty supporting is that of women. We are covered with guilt if we take a stand on our own behalf. We believe we should always be putting our energies "out there" for those who need it more. Women are notorious for not recognizing and standing up for our own needs and, on those rare occasions when we do, we are quickly immobilized when anyone calls us selfish.

THERE'S NO **reason for us to feel guilty when we try to take care of ourselves. We can feel guilty if we want to, and it doesn't make sense.**

✺ September 19

BEING PRESENT TO THE MOMENT

What they took for inattentiveness was a miracle of concentration.

—Toni Morrison

Have you ever watched a cat stalk a bird? Every muscle, every tendon, every heartbeat is focused on the prey.

Have you ever watched a cat stretch after a nap? Every muscle, every tendon, every heartbeat is totally involved in the stretch.

Sometimes when we are totally concentrating on a task we may seem rude and inattentive. Yet we are wholly present. We are present to our moment of focus.

These moments of complete focus are magical moments and frequently are times when we experience the oneness with our Higher Power and the process of the universe. We are totally within ourselves, and we are totally beyond ourselves.

I REJOICE for the moments of total oneness. I am truly myself when within and beyond myself.

✵ September 20

INTEGRITY

Real integrity is doing the right thing, knowing that nobody's going to know whether you did it or not.

—Oprah Winfrey

But *you* know, and who could be more important? You're the one you are absolutely sure you will have to live with for the rest of your life. Someone will know and that someone is you. No one else could be as important when it comes to matters of integrity. We can get away with a lot when it comes to others. But hopefully we are not so out of touch with ourselves that we can get away with anything with ourselves.

One of the pitfalls of doing too much and stretching ourselves too thin is opening the door for a slippage of our integrity. We feel so tired. We feel so strung out. Surely just this little shortcut won't matter. And it does. It matters to us. We might get away with it with others, and we know. We know, and it eats away at our souls.

That long-distance call on the office phone. That unkept promise to our family. That little bit of unnecessary gossip. That failure to report income. We know.

WE ARE much too precious to tamper with our integrity. Being alive is a special kind of bravery.

CLARITY

> *Women know a lot of things they don't read in the news-*
> *papers. It's pretty funny sometimes, how women know a*
> *lot of things and nobody can figure out how they know*
> *them.*
>
> —Meridel LeSueur

What a struggle it has been for us to repress our knowing for all these years . . . for all these centuries. We have ignored our own wisdom so that we fit more easily into the world around us.

How often have we kept our mouths shut at board meetings and staff meetings because sharing our knowledge would arouse a great hue and cry, or be completely ignored?

We have tried so hard to fit into a society that we did not create and to become acceptable to that society that we have become the amazing shrinking women. Yet, we know and we know we know.

THE WORLD **needs our knowledge and our wisdom. Our companies need our clarity. Our families need our clarity. We need our clarity.**

✢ September 22

CONFUSION

I seem to have an awful lot of people inside me.
                                    —Dame Edith Evans

Frequently it is the people that we carry around inside us who encourage our workaholism, our busyness and our careaholism.

We have little voices in our minds that tell us, "You are expendable. Employers can get rid of people who are not high producers. You are what you do. If you aren't doing something, you are nothing. No one will ever want you just for who you are. You have to make yourself indispensable, and then you can feel secure. You aren't intelligent *enough*. You're *too* intelligent." Voices, voices, voices.

No wonder we often feel confused. We have a chorus on twenty-four-hour duty.

GROWING UP and claiming our own lives is partially a process of listening to our own voices and distinguishing them from the crowd inside us, especially when the internal committee is a group of people who aren't very healthy.

❧ September 23

BECOMING THE CHANGE

*Become the change you want to see—those are the words
I live by.*

—Oprah Winfrey

Let's stop for a moment (I know that's a lot to ask!
Just try it anyway!) and let ourselves see what changes
we would like to see.

Whew! What a stopper! We can grumble about not
liking what is and start examining what changes we
would like to see?

Let's start with an easy one. Let's say we would like to
be appreciated more for what we do. Okay. How can we
"become" that?

Let's say we would like to get more rest. How can we
"become" ourselves getting more rest?

And what about having more time for ourselves?
Does that one make the list? How can we "become" that
change?

Then there's world peace. What can we do to
"become" world peace—a more peaceful person?

LIVING OUR wishes—living our changes—may require
something major. Are we ready for this?

✥ September 24

NURTURING RELATIONSHIPS

It takes two to destroy a marriage.

—Margaret Trudeau

And it takes those two and many others to make a marriage thrive.

It's very difficult to have a marriage—a real marriage—between two people who do too much or even with one person who does too much. Overworking, being too busy, and rushing around are very hard on a marriage. Bless our hearts, we do the best we can, and like Ursula Le Guin says, "Love doesn't just sit there like a stone; it has to be made, like bread, remade all the time, made new."

We can't fix something, then use it and expect it to stay fixed. We can't take the important things for granted and give our energy to the little things and expect the important ones to be there when we have the energy to notice. Human beings don't work very well that way, and relationships don't work at all that way.

WHAT HAVE you done recently to nurture the relationships that are important to you?

❧ September 25

CONFUSED THINKING

Every time you don't follow your inner guidance, you feel a loss of energy, loss of power, a sense of spiritual deadness.

—Shakti Gawain

Sometimes we just think too much. We have a problem to solve, and we believe that if we just can figure it out we will be all right. The more we figure, the more confused we become, until we have ourselves in a complete muddle. Then we use this occasion to beat ourselves up for being so dumb and stupid that we can't figure out the solution—and the downward spiral continues. We are indeed experiencing a loss of energy, a loss of power, a sense of spiritual deadness. We need to call upon some of our powers other than thinking. We need to "wait with" knowing.

STOP!! It's time to wait with our "inner guidance." It's always there. We have just covered it over with the compacted concentration of mental masturbation.

EXCELLENCE

My second favorite household chore is ironing; my first is hitting my head on the top bunk until I faint.

—Erma Bombeck

Housework is always fair game for humor. Maybe it's because down deep most of us still believe it's a woman's realm. Why is that? This particular belief seems to go right to our DNA.

I remember back in the heyday of the women's movement, hearing a woman talk about housecleaning. Her point was that girls had to *learn* how to clean house. Housecleaning wasn't a sex-linked gene. If women learned it, men could learn it. I tucked that one away for future use.

Then, several years ago, I had to admit that I was terrible at cleaning the house. I could clean up the kitchen and it looked worse! Then we discovered, quite by accident of course, that my husband was great at it. He's a Scandinavian. Talk about cleaning genes. He has them! I'm great with handling money and paying the bills and taxes. Why not have each of us do what we're good at? He doesn't like cleaning house much, but then, I don't like paying the bills and doing the taxes either. It works.

Once my husband started doing the housework, it wasn't nearly such fair game for humor.

IT'S GREAT **when we get over our brainwashing and can just do what we're good at.**

❧ September 27

HONORING SELF/PANIC/
CHOICES/SUPPORT

The place where I work is supposed to be a place that heals people, and it violates the people who work there.

— Rosie

We have been hearing more and more about unhealthy buildings and their effect upon our lives. However, as many of us begin to be aware and start to take better care of ourselves, we discover that our workplaces not only do not support our quest to become healthier, they actively interfere with it.

We find ourselves feeling frightened and overwhelmed. Are we going to have to give up our jobs to be healthy? Are we going to have to give up our journey into health in order to maintain our jobs? Neither option is too attractive.

Luckily, we do not have to make either of these choices today. We *do* need to get support for our journey toward health, however. Hopefully, there are possibilities for this support within and outside of the work setting. Support is crucial for becoming more whole.

I WILL **look around and open myself to as yet undiscovered sources of support wherever they are available.**

❧ September 28

LET'S DREAM

Behind every successful woman is a cleaner and a nanny.
—Anonymous

I used to hear some women say that they really wanted a wife. I don't want a wife, I want a *staff!* If I just had a wife, she would be as exhausted as I am.

We're not just talking about multi-tasking here. We're talking about a staff with full-time jobs.

Let's see—what do we need? Well, of course, a live-in nanny to help with the children and fill in on the car-pool/bus driver routes. Then a house cleaner—live-in, if possible, so that cooking healthy, gourmet meals to our specifications is part of the job. Then a personal assistant (P.A. the celebs call them—I could be a celeb; that's okay) to handle all the business things, appointments, movie schedules, perhaps with travel agent and best friend skills. Then a driver, so we can work—make notes for books and enjoy the scenery while in the car. Then—as long as we're dreaming—a masseuse one to seven days a week at home so we can stay relaxed and healthy after we do our exercise and have a soak. Oh yes, a handy person to handle the property and cars so we don't have to do that. Throw in an accountant, financial advisor, and tax consultant, and then, perhaps, I could get my work done.

ISN'T **dreaming great?**

✸ September 29

BUSYNESS/FRIENDSHIP

What a new idea! I had this friend who came to visit and it dawned on me . . . I didn't have to do anything.

—Mary

We busyaholics cannot even imagine the possibility of not having to *do* something. When a friend comes to visit, we rush around getting things in order, arranging, and preparing so they will feel welcome and have a good time.

We are so busy *before* they arrive that we are exhausted *when* they arrive. Or we keep ourselves so busy making them comfortable that we do not get to sit and be with them.

Somewhere in our busy little beings it is inconceivable that they can care for themselves and they just wanted to be with *us*.

TODAY **I have the possibility to be open to the possibility that someone who reaches out just wants to be with *me*.**

❧ September 30

FEAR/WORK

Know that it is good to work. Work with love and think of liking it when you do it. It is easy and interesting. It is a privilege. There is nothing hard about it but your anxious vanity and fear of failure.

—Brenda Ueland

Our work and the ability to do our work are gifts we have. Doing our work is so simple. We just do it. Our work is not difficult, confounding, or complicated. We make it that way sometimes. When we are able to focus on our work and just get down to it and do it one step at a time, it gets done and it usually gets done well. When we overwhelm ourselves by seeing only the totality of it looming before us and do not break it down into its smaller components, we begin to feel inadequate and incapable of completing the task. We then procrastinate as our anxiety and fears click into gear.

WHEN I TAKE my work one step at a time it is easy. Luckily, I can only do one step at a time anyway.

❧ October 1

To believe in something not yet proved and to underwrite it with our lives: it is the only way we can leave the future open.

—Lillian Smith

There once was a woman who said that she experienced the idea of Living in Process as akin to jumping off a cliff. Sometime after making that statement she related a dream in which she had come to the edge of a cliff and was aware of being very fearful of something coming up behind her. In the dream, she felt that she had only one positive choice—to jump off the cliff, which she did with great terror. Suddenly she was aware of a wonderful floating feeling. She opened her eyes and realized that her skirt had become a parachute: she was safe and floating comfortably.

"Leaving the future open" may be one of the most important commitments we make with our lives. Believing in something not yet proved may just be believing in ourselves.

WE NEVER know what will make good parachutes. When one is leaving the future open, it helps to know that there are parachutes not of our making in our lives.

❧ October 2

We grow neither better or worse as we get old, but more like ourselves.

—Mary Lamberton Becker

I once met a woman in her sixties who shared what a marvelous revelation it was to her to become completely gray. "I can just put my ideas out the way I want to," she said, "and I don't get all of that strange sexual energy from men coming at me like I did when I was younger."

Another woman in her fifties confided that one of the best-kept secrets in this culture was what she called "post-menopausal zest." "I thought I was a whiz before menopause," she whispered conspiratorially, "and you should see me now."

These were obviously women who had chosen to let process of aging facilitate their becoming more fully themselves.

AS THE DEMANDS to falsify ourselves lessen, we can more easily concentrate on being the person we have always been.

❧October 3

FEELING CRAZY

You were once wild here. Don't let them tame you!
—Isadora Duncan

We feel so overwhelmed by our feelings sometimes that we just feel like screaming. Women (and men!) do scream. We scream at our children, we scream at our spouses, we scream at our friends, and we scream at our employees. Often we and they attribute this behavior to the "time of the month" and write it off as crazy hormonal behavior. Down deep we feel ashamed, guilty, crazy, and unclean about this show of emotions.

Sometimes screaming is normal and necessary. We need to cry. We need to scream. It is part of our process and a normal response to living in a high-pressure, addictive society. However, we need *not* to scream at others. We need to have our safe places where we can let our feelings out: have a good cry or have a good scream. This processing is normal for the human organism. We just believed that we were the only ones who needed it.

WHEN I let my feelings out on others, I feel bad. When I just let my feelings out in a safe place, I feel good.

❧October 4

FREEDOM

> *Sisterhood, like female friendship, has at its core the affirmation of freedom.*

> —Mary Daly

For women to be truly friends, we have to shed the suspicious competitiveness toward one another that we have been trained into. We have to move beyond seeing other women as competitors for the "goodies" (males and male validation and attention). We have to be open to the possibility that *because* we are women we have mutual concerns and experiences that we need to share. To do this, we have to be willing to move beyond our training and education for separateness, to leap the chasm and become free to be ourselves with one another.

Once we have made the leap, we find a richness and depth in our female friendships that simply is not possible with men. We find ourselves saying again and again, "I know," "I know." It is in "affirming our freedom" from old brainwashing that we move into friendship and sisterhood.

THOUGH I HAVE been told otherwise, I need friends who are women.

❧October 5

MOVING MEDITATIONS

I'm not going to vacuum 'til Sears makes one you can ride on.

—Roseanne Barr

I hate vacuuming! It's one of those mindless activities that I have not been able to turn into a meditation.

I love the idea of a riding vacuum. I asked for and received a riding mower one Christmas—and then the men started mowing the grass. Do you think that will happen if I get a riding vacuum? Just a thought.

Seriously, one of the wonderful surprises about those repetitive little routine tasks is that we can secretly and surreptitiously turn them into movement meditations. Like cleaning the stove—I *love* cleaning the stove. I don't have to fight anyone to do it. It's not high on the popularity list. Rarely, if ever, has anyone joined me in stove-cleaning or even offered to join me.

So, there I am—cloths, sponges, cleaning liquids, and fingernails (the best tools!) in hand (no pun intended!)—alone, on my own, with as much as an hour (if I work slowly) of pure meditation alone time . . . not bad for a gal who does too much.

WE CAN TURN **almost anything into something it didn't look like it was—moving meditation.**

❧ October 6

OUR SANITY

> *What is my proudest accomplishment? I went through some pretty difficult times, and I kept my sanity.*
> —Jacqueline Kennedy Onassis

Keeping our sanity may be one of the greatest challenges a woman faces, especially women who do too much—and most women do too much.

Most of us don't have to face the level of difficult times that Jackie Kennedy had to face. Maybe that is why she is so admired and respected.

Yet, all of us have to face difficult times. There is no need to put a measurement on difficulty or to compare ourselves with Jacqueline. Difficult times are difficult times, and we all have to face them no matter who we are.

To keep our sanity—there's the challenge! Rarely do we get the support we really need. Rarely does anyone *really* understand what it is like for us and what we are truly going through. Rarely is there not someone or something that tells us that we are not doing it right.

Still, we persevere. We make it. We emerge with sanity intact (most times).

OUR SANITY is precious and much more resilient than we ever believed it could be.

❧ October 7

BEING PRESENT TO THE MOMENT

> *Miracles are unexpected joys, surprising coincidences, unexplainable experiences, astonishing beauties . . . absolutely anything that happens in the course of my day, except that at this moment I'm able to recognize its special value.*
>
> —Judith M. Knowlton

Miracles are constantly occurring around us. Serendipities abound in daily life.

The issue is not that these miracles are absent. The issue is that often *we* are absent. We are standing on a hill of diamonds, and we are looking for the gold mine beyond the next ridge.

As we reclaim ourselves, we begin to notice the extraordinariness of the ordinary. We quit *thinking* about being present and we start doing it.

THANK GOODNESS I have walked in circles long enough to wear the soles of my shoes so thin that the diamonds on which I stand can now get my attention.

❧ October 8

INDISPENSABLE/CONTROL

> *A few years ago, had someone called me an Indispensable Woman, I would have said, "Thank you." I would have considered it a compliment. Today, I know better.*
>
> —Ellen Sue Stern

As women who are caretakers and overworkers, we have often believed that we are indispensable. We have even made ourselves indispensable and then felt exhausted but secure. We believed that if the company, our children, our spouses, and our friends could not get along without us that there would always be a place for us in their lives. Our little hearts glowed when someone said, "What would I do without you?"

Thank goodness it is possible to teach an old dog new tricks! Many of us have seen that our indispensability not only was destructive to us, it was destroying all our relationships. We began to notice an undertone of resentment in those around us. People always resent those on whom they are dependent and those who try to control their lives.

I AM SO relieved that I discovered that being indispensable was killing me and my relationships. Now I have options!

❧ October 9

DESPAIR

> *A vacuum can only exist, I imagine, by the things that enclose it.*
>
> —Zelda Fitzgerald

A vacuum isn't just emptiness. It is the absence of something, and if it were not encased in its walls, a vacuum would not be possible.

We are familiar with the feeling of emptiness. There have been many times when we have felt that there just wasn't a drop of energy left in us. These periods are the "dark night of the soul." We will do anything to avoid feeling them; we even use whatever helps us *not* to feel.

We have been trapped by the very lives we have designed. Our architectural wonders have become prefabricated horrors. Our enclosures are of our own making, and only we can dismantle them.

JUST REMEMBER, when a vacuum is opened up, many interesting possibilities rush in.

❧ October 10

CONFUSION

She's half-notes scattered without rhythm.
—Ntozake Shange

We know that our lives have the potential of being a unique melody, and often they feel like "half-notes scattered without rhythm." When did the melody of our life go sour? Was it when we began to schedule more than we could handle? Was it when we began having difficulty relaxing? Was it when we began to feel resentful about the tasks we had agreed to do?

Sometime, probably gradually, our lives moved from concerto to crisis. The more we slip into this disease of doing too much, the more confused we become.

It is comforting to know that this confusion is something I use to cloud my thinking so I won't have to act.

WHEN I SEE my confusion as something I create, I have the possibility to let it go for a more productive coping mechanism.

❧ October 11

MONOTONE MIND

I don't want to get to the end of my life and find that I just lived the length of it. I want to have lived the width of it as well.

—Diane Ackerman

When we become overly focused on our work, our children, our homes, or our relationships, we become one-dimensional women. Throughout history, and more recently with the women's movement, we have been painfully aware that women have often been limited to the more mindless tasks of the society.

Unfortunately, as more of us break in to the ranks of the privileged (as we have viewed them), we again find that we have the opportunity to become dull and narrow . . . just in a different way. The content has changed. The process remains the same.

In order to reclaim our souls, we need to recognize that width is as important as length in the living of our days.

WIDTH ADDS **a dimension to length. Depth adds a dimension to both length and width. The world is at least three-dimensional.**

CONFUSED THINKING/JUDGMENTALISM

> *I realize what a lot of negativity there is in the world and all around us, and how easy it is to become part of that negativity and to be sucked into it and become part of the chaos and confusion if one isn't very careful.*
>
> —Eileen Caddy

Negativity is one aspect of typical confused thinking. In our work lives, we are rewarded for analyzing, comparing, criticizing, and being negative. It is easy to see how we become sucked into negativity and the focus upon what's wrong. The key here is judgmentalism.

I was a keynote speaker at a convention once. One of the other keynote speakers came up to me and told me how much she just *loved Women's Reality*. She said it really had spoken to her soul.

Then, when she gave her presentation, she ripped *Women's Reality* to shreds. I was shocked and asked her why she did it. "I'm a teacher at an Ivy League college," she said. "If you don't rip things to shreds, no one respects you."

It's important to see what's wrong in any situation and what needs to be changed. When judgmentalism enters in, however, the observation takes on a tone of negativity, and that negativity is very seductive.

LEARNING to see clearly and not get sucked into confusion and negativity is one of the challenges every day of our lives.

❧ October 13

CONTROL

When nothing is sure, everything is possible.
—Margaret Drabble

These words strike terror in the heart of the woman who does too much. Even the prospect of admitting that nothing is sure stimulates our minds to get very busy listing the things in our lives that we are sure about. When we are honest, the list is very small: death is perhaps the only really *sure* thing. Everything else is merely possible.

One of the exciting wonders of recognizing our need for control and beginning to let it go is the weightlessness of the anticipation that everything is possible. When we realize we don't know, we are open to what we don't know.

LIVING by faith is flying by the seat of my pants. I'm really living that way anyway, but I have denied it as long as I could.

❧ October 14

FEELING OVERWHELMED

> *I feel like I'm fighting a battle when I didn't start a war.*
> —Dolly Parton

Sometimes we feel overwhelmed with forces outside ourselves. We find ourselves embroiled in family or organizational wars and infighting that we do not believe we started and that we certainly do not want to participate in. Yet once in them we feel as if we have to fight, or at least try to stop them.

Both behaviors feed such battles. The one thing we have the power to decide about is our participation. We have the power to decide *not* to participate. It is amazing how battles dissipate when no one participates. When we feel overwhelmed by the battle, we cannot see or we forget that we have the power of nonparticipation.

We need to pull back to see the option of nonparticipation.

NONPARTICIPATION **may be one of the most powerful tools we have—peace tools, that is.**

BEAUTY

> *Because the best way to know the truth or beauty is to try*
> *to express it. And what is the purpose of existence here or*
> *yonder but to discover truth and beauty and express it,*
> *i.e., share it with others?*
>
> —Brenda Ueland

If the purpose of existence is to discover truth and beauty and share our discovery with others, some of us may have been on the wrong track.

In our need to achieve and move ahead, we have become stingy. We have come to believe that there is a limited amount of power and success and that if we give anything away, we will have less. So we develop the wonderful defect of stinginess.

We have begun to think that if we share ideas or awareness, others will steal them. We censor, copyright, choke our knowledge, and . . . we lose.

GREAT IDEAS **belong to everyone. It is only the small ones that have to be counted.**

✤ October 16

OUR CHILDREN

And then you have football practice. I leave work at 5:05 when we shut down. Then I backtrack the bus route—I pick up the little one, I pick up the big one. I change clothes at the babysitter's 'cause I don't have time to go home and we have football practice at 6:00. Then we sit for an hour and a half or two hours. Then we run to McDonald's. Then we run home and into the bath, read the homework, and go to bed. That's my life.

—Lucinda

This woman has an executive business position. It's not that her job is "unimportant" so she should do all the running. She is not a single mother. Yet, like so many women, it seems she has all the responsibility for the children. I wondered about the hour and a half with the little one while her son practiced football. Is this the time she has with the little one? I doubt that it's "down time" for her or quality time for either of them.

What are we doing to our children? Are we *raising* our children? Do we get to know our children? Do they get to know us? Why do we have children?

THERE ARE **many questions we need to ask and answer about our lives.**

❧ October 17

BEAUTY/ONENESS/AWE

> *Since you are like no other being ever created since the
> beginning of time, you are incomparable.*
>
> —Brenda Ueland

When I read those words of Brenda Ueland, I take a deep breath and let it out very slowly. I am incomparable. Just letting myself truly know that elicits a feeling of awe and reverence . . . reverence for myself.

In Twelve-Step circles there is a concept of "terminal uniqueness." One is terminally unique when one believes that no one else has had it so bad and that we are the center of the universe. When we insist in defining the world from our own perspective, we are operating out of terminal uniqueness. Terminal uniqueness erodes the soul.

When we accept and celebrate our uniqueness, we take our place in the universe.

THERE ARE **many things of beauty, and I am one of them!**

✤ October 18

There are no new truths, but only truths that have been recognized by those who have perceived them without noticing.

—Mary McCarthy

Our greatest learnings often come when we are unaware that we are learning something. We can study a technique or focus upon a project for days, and the truth or the essence of it just does not seem to click. Then something happens. The fog clears and we notice that we have moved to a new level of truth without ever knowing how we got there. It was not our straining or trying that brought us to this new level. It was our willingness to be aware of what had already taken place that opened new doors.

The most important processes of our being are best perceived by noticing. They are fed to us from somewhere beyond us.

TODAY **has the potential to be a day in which I can recognize the deep truths working within me.**

❧ October 19

KNOWING WHEN TO LET GO

> *In the end, it's probably not the holding on that will summarize our lives. It is the letting go that will be of the greater significance.*
>
> —Anne Wilson Schaef

Letting go is no easy process, especially for women who do too much. After all, haven't we made our reputation with our tenacity, our stubbornness, and our ability to persevere against tremendous odds?

One of the fallouts of doing too much is that we lose our perspective on what is important and what isn't. We lose the ability to discern what is a little battle and not worth our effort and what is an important battle where we need to stand our ground.

We dissipate and squander our energies on little things that really don't matter that much and have nothing left when we need to face up to the really important.

This loss of our ability to discern the small from the large issues is one of the disasters of our doing too much.

WE NEED to be able to let go of the little things so we are there for the big ones. If we do that, we may discover there are many fewer big ones than we thought.

❧ October 20

AWARENESS OF PROCESS/CONTROL

Time is a dressmaker specializing in alterations.
—Faith Baldwin

We often think that we are "just about to get it together" when life gives us another opportunity for learning. Many of us have tried to treat our lives like our houses. We have believed that we could get our houses fixed up just the way we wanted them and then they would stay that way forever. We have felt personally attacked when slipcovers wear out, when a room needs to be repainted, or when an appliance breaks down. We have set up our lives based upon a static and wished-for universe. We have believed that once fixed things should stay fixed, whether they be our houses, our jobs, or ourselves. In trying to make ourselves and our universe static, we have set ourselves up for intense moments of frustration and failure. Our attempts to control the normal processes of life have taken their toll on us and those around us.

I AM a process. Life is a process. Alterations are a constant, integral part of the process.

✢ October 21

FEAR

> *While we wait in silence for that final luxury of fearless-ness, the weight of that silence will choke us.*
>
> —Audre Lorde

Our silence about the issues that matter most to us thunders in our heads and bodies like a galloping herd of buffalo. The canyons of our inner beings resound with our unspoken ideas and perceptions.

Our fear confines our souls in the daily holocausts of silent existence. Our fear is real. It is palpable. We can feel it. We must learn to honor it and move through it. We cannot deny it, and we cannot "wait . . . for that final luxury of fearlessness." To become fixated in our fear is to creep in to that choking silence that devours our soul. No woman must speak when she is not ready. We must respect one another in our silence. When we face our fears, we may hear our voices.

MY FEAR is real. I will honor it. And I do not need to live my life out of it.

BEING DIRECT

If you can't be direct, why be?

—Lily Tomlin

Being direct is almost archaic in this culture. With all the "spin," "handling," innuendo, and outright lying it is difficult to know what anyone is saying and what is real or not real.

"Feminine" women have been trained in smooth talk, inference, manipulation, and control. Our mothers and grandmothers were masters of the "soft sell." They had to be. They were raised to be impotent and dependent.

We often feel resentful and sad because we find ourselves dealing with illusion. It's not that we don't perceive reality. We do! We just don't want to have to dig it out all the time.

We women are good at seeing the whole picture. We are good at seeing the fine details. We are great at generating creative options. And we are excellent at understanding the emotional as well as the intellectual nuances.

As we women are changing and our roles are changing, do we want to slip into the male form of smooth talk and spin? We have some choices to make here. This particular choice may not seem like such a big one, but it has great implications.

WHY NOT **be direct? Being direct takes so much less time and energy. Why be if we can't be direct?**

❧ October 23

ACCEPTANCE/LIVING IN THE NOW

The opportunity of life is very precious and it moves very quickly.

—Ilyani Ywahoo

This is it! The life that is ours is the one we are living today. There is no other. The more we try to hold on to our illusions of what we *think* it is or what we think it *should* be, the less time and energy we have to live it.

How many times have we heard about people who worked hard and longed for the day when retirement would come, only to drop dead just before or just after they retired? How fast it all went!

Our lives are so precious. Each moment has the possibility of a new discovery. Yet when it passes, that moment never returns.

ONLY AS I AM aware of and to the best of my ability living the present will I have the opportunity to *do* my life and not just pass through it.

PARENTING

> *If we try to control and hold on to our children, we lose them. When we let them go, they have the option to return to us more fully.*
>
> —Anne Wilson Schaef

Few of us have a Ph.D. in parenting. If we did, we would probably be worse than we are now. How much energy we put into trying to mold and control our children, not for their sakes, but so they will reflect better on us.

We are unable to see them as separate and important beings who are here to share a time with us so that we can learn from each other. We think we *need* them to validate our lives and our choices in life. When we do that, we use them as objects, which is totally disrespectful to them and to ourselves.

TO LOVE our children is to see them, respect them, share life with them . . . and always to let go. And remember, letting go is totally different from abandoning.

❧ October 25

HOPES AND DREAMS

Hope is the thing with feathers
That perches in the soul . . .
And sings the tune without words
And never stops . . . at all

—Emily Dickinson

It is nice to remember that we have a little feathered being deep in us that sings unceasingly.

So often, we believe that we have come to a place that is void of hope and void of possibilities, only to find that it is the very hopelessness that allows us to hit bottom, give up our illusion of control, turn it over, and ask for help. Out of the ashes of our hopelessness comes the fire of our hope.

To be without hopes and dreams is a place of loss . . . loss of our birthright as a human being. Hope does spring and sing eternal, even when we have wax in our ears.

BY RECOGNIZING **and affirming my feelings of hopelessness, I open the possibility to move into the hope that does, indeed, pass all understanding. Hope is a process of the soul, not the brain.**

❧ October 26

> We were pulled along by our version of a (medical) cen-
> ter where women could come to have their bodies cared
> for and have their innermost thoughts and beliefs lis-
> tened to, a center where women's wisdom would be cul-
> tivated and celebrated.
>
> But after two years we noticed that the old familiar
> patterns of burnout and exhaustion were inexorably
> creeping into our lives.
>
> —Christiane Northrup

Wherever we go—there we are. Just because we move
to a new location and try to set up a place where our
hopes and dreams can blossom doesn't mean that our
dreams will come true.

When I used to do organizational consulting, we
talked about the phenomenon of "form as a fix." Organizations believed that if they just changed locations and
developed a new organizational structure everything
would be all right. They believed if the forms changed
then everything else would follow. Not true. Many
organizations go through one structural change after
another and nothing really changes.

We forget that organizations are made up of people
and unless the people change, the organizations will just
be stuck in old or new ruts. Yet, change is possible.

NEW STARTS **start from within.**

❧ October 27

CREATIVITY

> *It is the creative potential itself in human beings that is the image of God.*
>
> —Mary Daly

What a beautiful way to think of our creativity! If we do not express our creativity, we are blocking the potential of the flowing energy of the image of God.

For most women who do too much, creativity has a very low place in our list of priorities. We don't have time to be creative. We will be creative later (and later . . . and later). We don't really believe in *our* creativity. Only special women have real creativity, and we are so terrified that we may not be one of these women that we won't even try to see what *our* creativity is. After all, "If you can't do something outstanding, it's better not to do anything at all."

WHEN I think of my creative potential as the "image of God," within me(!), I feel a deep, profound, and intense awe.

❧ October 28

COMMUNICATION

> *The only listening that counts is that of the talker who*
> *alternately absorbs and expresses ideas.*
>
> —Agnes Repplier

Women have historically been good listeners. We have been trained to listen carefully and even to "listen with the third ear." Caretakers need to listen, often not saying what they think they need to say.

As we have become women who do too much, we find our listening skills on the wane. We cut people off in the middle of sentences. We assume we know what an employee is going to say, and we act on that assumption. We even become enamored with the sound of our own voice.

We must remember that communication is more than a monologue. Good communication is a balance of speaking and sharing, listening carefully, and absorbing before we speak again.

We as women often limit ourselves to listening or talking. Thus we miss the meaning of communication.

TODAY **I have the opportunity to observe if I practice all three aspects of communication.**

✤ October 29

ONENESS

> *To the Indian mind, the life of the universe has not been analyzed, classified, and a great synthesis formed of the parts. To him [sic] the varied forms are equally important and varied.*

—Alice C. Fletcher

Recently, I heard a woman discussing why she enjoyed spending part of her time with an elderly woman friend in a household of women. "Everything gets done so easily," she said. "All the jobs have equal status. Washing the clothes or cooking a meal has just as much status as the work we do in our offices as physicians. It all just flows."

I was reminded of how much we analyze our universe, assign random values, and chop up our lives. That process not only makes our lives more difficult, it alienates us from the experience of oneness with all things, and without that experience, we don't know that we belong.

WHEN I DIMINISH **others' belongingness in the universe,** *my* **belongingness becomes uncertain.**

❧ October 30

BEING OBSESSED/NEEDING OTHERS

She who rides a tiger is afraid to dismount.

—Proverb

Being obsessed with our work is often thought to be a requirement for success. Yet, when was it that the tail started wagging the dog? Where was the point at which we stopped doing our work, and it began doing us?

It is a lot harder to get off the roller coaster in the middle than it was to get on it. This is why we need the companionship of others who are struggling with the same issues: they support our process of getting unhooked from our obsessive doing.

It is only with the support of others and the renewed connection with a power greater than ourselves that we can hope to become whole.

I SUPPOSE I can dismount if I have a few people helping to hold the tiger. I have been known to dismount!

❧ October 31

BEING PROJECTLESS

How beautiful it is to do nothing, and then rest afterward.

—Spanish proverb

For many of us the thought of doing nothing is terrifying. We cannot imagine what life would be like if we were not slaving away at our projects. Not to have our projects waiting for us is like trying to live with parts missing. We have become so dependent upon the security of the next project that they are no longer *our* projects. We are owned by them.

Workaholics often experience some depression when they complete a task. Instead of dealing with the completely natural and often feared feeling of letdown, we overlap the completion with the beginning of a new project. Hence, we never have to deal with separation or beginnings and endings. In fact, we never have to deal with anything except our exhaustion. In fact, we never have to deal with anything.

PERHAPS TODAY I could experiment with doing nothing, and resting afterward.

❧ November 1

WORK/CAUSES

Beware of people carrying ideas. Beware of ideas carry-
ing people.

—Barbara Grizzuti Harrison

Ideas can be so seductive, and we are so easily seduced. We forget that ideas are just that, abstractions that have been thought up.

We often lose ourselves in ideas and become so caught up in them that we cannot distinguish between ourselves and the idea. When we reach this level of enmeshment with our ideas, we experience any attack on our ideas as an attack on our being.

Being so attached to our ideas often results in a widening gap between what we are espousing and what we actually do. How often we kill in the name of love. We talk about cooperation and we try to force it on others. We get an idea for high productivity and we interfere with productivity by demanding an adherence to our idea. We start out carrying an idea and soon it is carrying us.

I WILL NOT let what I think destroy what I believe.

❧ November 2

GUILT

Who I am is what I have to give. Quite simply, I must remember that's enough.

—Anne Wilson Schaef

Often, when we look in our inner recesses, we feel that we are lacking. We have been a disappointment to others. We couldn't "be there" when we should have been, and we didn't have all the information we should have had. Somehow, though it may be just a vague feeling, we have failed.

It appears that feeling guilty is a sex-linked gene. There seems to be an infinitely close connection between feeling guilty and being female.

When we feel guilty, we try to make up for what we have or have not done. We feel we need to "make something special," to make things all right. We need to make up for a "transgression" even if we don't know what it was.

I CANNOT make up for something I think I haven't done or have done wrong by trying to make others or myself feel guilty.

❧ November 3

CRISIS ORIENTATION

> *The Physician says I have "Nervous*
> *prostration."*
> *Possibly I have—I do not know the names of*
> *sickness. The crisis*
> *of the sorrow of so many years is all that*
> *tires me.*

> —Emily Dickinson

Physicians have invented many erudite and confounding names for women who work themselves into a complete frazzle. We spend our lives moving from one crisis to another. As a matter of fact, we have become so competent at handling crisis that we feel most at home in the middle of one. If the truth were known, we women who do too much often create a crisis when things are going smoothly. When things are quiet, we keep waiting for the other shoe to fall and we feel relieved when we have a crisis to be managed. We know how to do that.

SERIAL CRISES are exciting, *and* they are exhausting. I don't want crisis to be the origin of yet another medical label nor do I want the "sorrow of so many years" to weigh me down.

❧ November 4

FIXERS AND FIXEES

> *Once again I was brought to my knees as I learned that*
> *each of us must access inner wisdom for herself. I can*
> *point out the road map, perhaps, but I must completely*
> *let go of the outcome.*
>
> —Christiane Northrup

We live in a society of "experts" and people looking for experts. Unfortunately, the two groups fit together quite nicely. Also unfortunately, the "fit" never works. This dysfunction causes problems on both sides.

The "fixers" really want to have the answers. They love the glow of "expert" and most do sincerely want to be of help. The power in the role is quite seductive, especially when so many are begging them to have the answers.

The "to be fixed" desperately want to believe that someone—anyone—must have the answers because they know they don't. And, what a risk it is to be responsible for themselves when they are so sure that they don't know what they need to know.

And so the dance continues.

WHAT A TERRIFYING RELIEF it is when we run into someone who gives us information—even a road map—and completely lets go of the outcome, knowing that there are other road maps and other information that may also be important.

FINANCIAL SECURITY

It seems that the rewards of an affluent society turn bitter as gall in the mouth.

—Natalie Shaeness

An affluent society often functions as a giant tranquilizer. In the pursuit of the rewards of affluence, we have to tune out our awareness so completely that we become destructive to our bodies and our psyches. We have to develop addictions to shut off our awareness of what is *really* important to us. We operate out of denial and are threatened by anyone wanting to challenge our head-in-the-sand approach.

When we see the sole purpose of our work as the pursuit of affluence, we have lost track of ourselves and what is meaningful work for us. Our spiritual selves have become an abstraction, if they exist at all.

IF I SPEND my life pursuing things that ultimately have little meaning to me, I run the risk of feeling that I have wasted my life. I have enough risks I'm running without that one.

❧ November 6

The shortest answer is doing.

—English proverb

Although we women who do too much do overwork and overextend ourselves, we also struggle with procrastination. Just let a deadline approach, and we slip in to the sloughs of lethargy. We just can't get ourselves going. Working at a steady pace is not our style. We work in spurts: intense crisis-mode operating and then nothing. Just thinking about deadlines exhausts us. Meeting them wipes us out.

Deadlines are a threat to women who do too much. They offer us an opportunity to slip back into our old patterns. And, we know old patterns can kill us. Remember, relapse is just as dangerous for a workaholic as it is for an alcoholic. We both have a progressive, fatal disease.

Deadlines offer us the opportunity to reach out and ask for support.

THIS DEADLINE is a gift to help me see how much progress I have made and how I can function differently.

INTUITION

> *What I am actually saying is that we each need to let our intuition guide us, and then be willing to follow that guidance directly and fearlessly.*

> —Shakti Gawain

One of the most frightening things in the world is to trust our intuition and follow that trusting. It is hard for us to believe that what the Quakers call our "inner light" is really the way our power greater than ourselves speaks most clearly to us.

When we are one with ourselves and our process, we are truly one with the process of the universe. When we are one with ourselves, our lives seem to fall into place effortlessly. All of us know the feeling of moments of effortless living. When we have the courage to trust our intuition, life begins to live itself.

MY INTUITION **connects me with the voice I need to hear.**

❧ November 8

ACTION

There is really nothing more to say—except why. But since why is difficult to handle, one must take refuge in how.

—Toni Morrison

There are often events in our lives that just do not make sense. In spite of our best efforts, projects fail. It is important to take stock of the situation and accept our part in the failure and then move on.

When we get stuck on the why, we can stay stuck for a long time. We so want to understand, and it is so difficult to admit that some things just make no sense. Remember, "Whying is dying."

Faith in living does not ask why. Faith in living asks how and does it.

THE EVENT may not be the problem. Our need to understand it may be the problem.

❧ November 9

HANGING IN/STUBBORNNESS

It is not true that life is one damn thing after another . . .
it's the same damn thing over and over again.

—Edna St. Vincent Millay

Our inner process gives us every opportunity to learn what we need to learn. Our inner being is very conservation-minded—it continues to recycle our stuff, and recycle our stuff, and recycle our stuff. If we don't get the lesson the first time around, we get another chance . . . and another . . . and another. Life gives us every opportunity to work through whatever we need to work through.

Unfortunately, every time an opportunity for learning recycles, it comes with a greater and greater force. The intensity of the force with which we have to be hit is directly related to our denial, stubbornness, and illusion of control. Life will cycle the same damn thing over and over again, until we get it.

We're lucky that way.

I'M GLAD my inner process hangs in with me. Sometimes I'm a slow learner.

❧ November 10

LETTING GO/CONTROL

The true secret of giving advice is, after you have honestly given it, to be perfectly indifferent whether it is taken or not and never persist in trying to set people right.
—Hannah Whitall Smith

Actually, we probably should never give advice, even when someone asks for it. However, it is often helpful to give information and then *let it go*. Too often we get invested in our information and are so sure of our rightness that we have to make certain the other person *accepts* it. Somehow, deep inside of us their acceptance of our information is directly tied to our self-worth. If they don't accept our advice and act on it, we are somehow not liked, respected, valued, and a whole string of other adjectives.

As we get healthier, we are learning to give and let go.

I HAVE good information to share. It is more likely to be heard when I give it and let it go.

LOVE

> *The story of a love is not important—what is important is that one is capable of love. It is perhaps the only glimpse we are permitted of eternity.*

> —Helen Hayes

All too often, we women who do too much confuse "falling in love" with loving. We like the "buzz," the intensity of the adrenaline rush of falling in love. It's exciting and "relieves us from the pressure of our overextended lives for a while." Even the excitement of fitting it into our busy schedules is titillating. And— eventually—it wears us out. We have become so inured to intensity that we need something new to give us our high.

Beware of instant intimacy. Beware of buzzing intensity. Both may be fun, and they are most likely not love. They are a by-product of the way we are living our lives.

Love is slower, deeper, and easier. Love takes us into and beyond ourselves, not just into our self-centeredness. Love is available to all of us. Yet, we may have to take some time to learn about love, because we haven't had many models around us who know how it's done.

WE ARE all capable of love whether we know it or not. To "glimpse that eternity" we may have to take the time to let go of old illusions and learn new ways of being.

CREATIVITY

> *As soon as I began painting what was in my head the*
> *people around me were shocked.*
>
> —Leonor Fini

Our creativity, once unleashed, knows no time or space. It is like a passionate lover that demands to be heard. No wonder we are so afraid of it. It can turn our world topsy-turvy. And maybe our worlds *need* to be turned topsy-turvy.

When our creativity shows itself, it is now. The ideas we are having now are a result of who we are now, our life situations now, and what is going on inside us now. We will not be the same women fifteen years from now.

Expressing our creativity now in whatever form it takes is a way of enriching our lives, making us more interesting women, and releasing the tension of not creating.

I OWE IT to myself to find time for my creative self.

❧ November 13

INSPIRATION

> *We need a new ethos of individual responsibility and caring—we have to summon up what we believe is morally and ethically and spiritually correct and do the best that we can with God's guidance.*
>
> —Hillary Rodham Clinton

We all need to be inspired. Inspiration not only points us to what is possible, it energizes us with what is possible for us.

When we are overworked, overextended, tired, and irritable, we don't have much room for inspiration. All we want to do is collapse, pull the proverbial covers over our head, and vegetate. We just want to put one foot in front of the other and trudge along as best we can, looking neither left or right, neither up or down, neither in or out.

Yet our trudging does not energize us. It does not give us life. It does not offer us the opportunity to gaze at the stars and become one with them.

Our morality, ethics, spirituality, and guidance from a power greater than ourselves give us energy.

WHAT INSPIRES you? What challenges you? What reconnects you to God's guidance?

❧ November 14

CONTROL

> *I was torn by two different time concepts. I knew which one made sense, but the other one was fighting hard for survival. [Structure, regimentation, orderedness. Which had absolutely nothing to do with anything.]*
>
> —Robyn Davidson

One of the ways we practice our illusion of control and protect our disease is to surround ourselves with people like ourselves who do the same things we do. When we are surrounded by women who also rush around, are always busy, work too much, and take care of everyone, we seem normal. Our way of doing things seems normal and even *right!* We avoid putting ourselves in situations where our control skills are not shared and valued, because then in that situation we might notice that we do not like controlling at all. Structure, regimentation, and orderedness are the way things have to be, or so we believe. That is why when we do allow ourselves to travel, we stay in American hotels with well-known names, if possible.

OUR ILLUSION **of control is more cunning than a cat, and it has more than nine lives.**

ACCEPTANCE

> *Now I think my point is that I have learned to live with it all . . . with being old . . . whatever happens . . . all of it.*
>
> —Edelgard

How wonderful that we not only have the opportunity to live our lives, we have the opportunity to *accept* them! We have spent so much time and energy foolishly fighting things that we cannot change and butting our heads up against steel-reinforced brick walls that we have not stopped to ask ourselves if this is the hill we want to die on.

Part of learning to live our lives is developing the ability to accept what cannot be changed and learn to live creatively with those situations. Also, we need to discover what can be challenged and to move forward with courage when necessary. Acceptance is not resignation. Acceptance is serenity embracing life.

TODAY **my life is enough just the way it is, *and* it is mine.**

❧ November 16

FEELING CRAZY AND COPING

> *Crazy and coping are interactive. They go together and*
> *are mutually supportive. When I'm crazy, I believe I*
> *have to cope and when I am trying to cope, I get crazy.*
> —Karen M.

The crazier we feel, the more we feel we should be able to cope. We lose our ability to make clear and sane judgments about ourselves and the situations in which we find ourselves. We find ourselves trying to accomplish feats that no sane person would even attempt and fully expecting that we should be able to accomplish them with great ease. In fact, our progressively taking on more and more is directly related to our creeping closer to the brink. It is difficult to tell which is the chicken and which is the egg—probably neither. They are interactive. Our taking on more and more drives us closer and closer to the brink and getting closer and closer to the brink results in our taking on more and more.

INERTIA **is the force that keeps an object at rest when at rest or in motion when in motion, unless acted upon by an external force.**

We have an inertia problem. We need an outside force. We can't do this by ourselves.

❧ November 17

SELF-AWARENESS

There's a period of life when we swallow a knowledge of ourselves and it becomes either good or sour inside.
—Pearl Bailey

Self-knowledge is always a good thing. No one else possesses the capacity to know us as well as we can know ourselves.

It is in the awareness of ourselves that our strength lies. And awareness of every aspect of ourselves allows us to become who we are.

Often our rejection of various aspects of ourselves keeps us stuck. Some of us quite readily see those aspects of our personalities that we perceive as negative and just as readily beat ourselves up for those characteristics. Others go to the other extreme and sugarcoat our self-perceptions, putting all blame and responsibility for who we have become on anyone and anything outside of ourselves. Neither approach is helpful or growth-producing.

IT IS ONLY in our self-awareness that we can taste the bitter and the sweet and grow into who we *can* be.

ACCEPTANCE/AMBITION

I long to accomplish a great and noble task, but it is my chief duty to accomplish small tasks as if they were great and noble.

—Helen Keller

Such amazing words from a person whose life in itself was such "a great and noble task"! In Helen Keller's words we sense such deep acceptance of her life. We have a glimmer of insight into the paradox that if we just take one step at a time and do each task as it presents itself, we may discover we have done great and noble things. If we are *trying* to do great and noble tasks, we may well find that we have missed those magic opportunities just to do what we need to do. God never gives us anything too big or too small for us. Our egos may need the small.

As the author Brenda Ueland says, "Try to discover your true, honest, untheoretical self." Our theoretical self often interferes with our real self.

MY ILLUSION **of myself may not be who I am. My illusion of my work may not be what it is.**

TIME MANAGEMENT

> *I'm working so hard on my time management that I
> don't get anything done.*
>
> —Anonymous

We can get so involved in a new technique that the
technique itself becomes another monster in our lives,
and we become slaves to it.

Time management can be a good thing. It can help
us look at how we spend our time. It can help us become
more efficient in getting a job done and can help us
learn new ways of doing old things. None of us is as efficient as we could be, and efficiency is useful.

However, when we use any technique to support our
workaholism, that technique becomes part of the problem. Unfortunately, we can use anything.

Hopefully, we will develop better perspectives for
evaluating our use of such tools to make our lives more
serene and healthy.

TOOLS **are for my use, not vice versa.**

APPRECIATION

> *You must not think that I feel, in spite of it having ended
> in such defeat, that my "life has been wasted" here, or
> that I would exchange it with that of anyone I know.*
> —Isak Dinesen

One of the most important aspects of our lives is that
they are *our* lives. No one else could live them exactly
the way we are living them. Everything that happens in
our lives is an opportunity for learning. Those moments
of frustration often turn into moments of joy and creativity.

What an extraordinary experience it is to look back
and truly feel that we can celebrate our lives—all of
them.

Returning to our spiritual selves provides a path to
appreciation.

I HAVE the opportunity to walk the path of appreciation
today. It is not possible that my life has been wasted. Defeat
is not waste unless I turn it into waste.

ALONE TIME

Women's normal occupations in general run counter to creative life or contemplative life or saintly life.
—Anne Morrow Lindbergh

There is not much in our lives that supports our creativity. Work in the home and work outside the home are generally not conducive to the kind of nurturing that every human being needs. As we buy into the workaholism, competitiveness, and stress of the dominant society, we find ourselves changing and losing many of the qualities that were most precious to us.

We have rebelled against and don't have time for women's work, and we have raced headlong into men's work. Now we not only get to do women's work, we get to do both and work twice as hard.

We find our moments of creative time or contemplative time, or even saintly time are few and far between. Yet, we need these times and we deserve these times for ourselves.

I WILL TRY to remember that when I take time for myself, I have much more to offer to myself, my work, and those around me.

WHOLENESS

Women's work is always toward wholeness.

—May Sarton

When we women do *our* work, we move toward wholeness. The world is in need of wholeness. The world is in need of women's way of working.

Too long we have doubted ourselves and tried to fit comfortably into a male modality. To have wholeness, we need to make our contribution too. To have wholeness, we need to know our values and value our knowing.

We have reneged on our responsibility to this society and this planet. It is time that we courageously put our thoughts, ideas, and values out there and let them stand for themselves.

WHEN I DO my work, is wholeness.

TURNING IT OVER

> *I need to take an emotional breath, step back, and remind myself who's actually in charge of my life.*
> —Judith M. Knowlton

How often we want to stop, turn around angrily, and shout, "*who's in charge here?*" We have tried to be in charge of our lives and have learned again and again that our being in charge has not quite worked. Sooooo . . . if we aren't, who is?

It seems too nebulous for a practical, professional woman just to step back and turn her life over to some vague power that may exist out there. Isn't religion for weaklings? Aren't those who want to depend upon a power greater than themselves just being dependent and not taking responsibility for themselves? Perhaps. Yet, when we think dualistically like that, when we grab the power or we give it up, we miss the point.

Life is a process of cooperating with the forces in our lives and living out that partnership.

WE ARE in charge together. Not as controllers . . . as a living process.

SOLITUDE

Like water which can clearly mirror the sky and the trees only so long as its surface is undisturbed, the mind can only reflect the true image of the Self when it is tranquil and wholly relaxed.

—Indra Devi

How often are our minds "tranquil and wholly relaxed?" Do we recognize that time for solitude is just as important to our work as keeping informed, preparing reports, or planning? As author Brenda Ueland says, "Presently your soul gets frightfully sterile and dry because you are so quick, snappy and efficient about doing one thing after another that you have no time for your own ideas to come in and develop and gently shine."

We have to give ourselves time. We have to give our ideas time. If we don't neither we nor they can gently shine, and we cannot hear the voice of our inner process speaking to us.

SOLITUDE **is not a luxury. It is a right and a necessity.**

❧ November 25

PERFECTIONISM

> *Don't try to be such a perfect girl, darling. Do the best you can without too much anxiety or strain.*
>
> —Jesse Barnard

How many of us have longed for words from our mothers like the ones Jesse Barnard wrote to her daughter. Perhaps, if our parents hadn't needed us to be perfect, *we* wouldn't need to be perfect. Unfortunately, even when others do not demand perfection of us, we who do too much demand it of ourselves.

We forget that when push comes to shove the only standard of perfection we have to meet is to be perfectly ourselves. Whenever we set up abstract, external standards and try to force ourselves to meet them, we destroy ourselves.

DOING THE BEST I can without too much anxiety or strain sounds like a relaxing way to live.

❧ November 26

RIGHT ON

I still have this enormous respect for what the human spirit can accomplish in a troubled time.

—Katie Couric

As if we didn't have enough to deal with! Now we have terrorists, politics, pollution, and the economy. When will it stop?

Probably never! Were there ever people who didn't believe that they lived in a troubled time? I doubt it.

The truth is—*This is it.* This is life. We can't keep using the "troubled times" smoke screen to justify not living our lives right now.

We have developed so many excuses for not dealing with the things that really matter to us until "later."

Well, later is right now. Right now is when we can accomplish what we want to accomplish. Right now is when we can enjoy our children. Right now is when we can relate to the people we love. Right now is when we can become the person we have always wanted to be.

WHATEVER IS IMPORTANT to us, we can start or do right now.

HAPPINESS

If you haven't been happy very young, you still can be happy later on, but it's much harder, you need more luck.

—Simone de Beauvoir

We all carry influences and experiences from our childhood into our adult lives. Dysfunctional families are the norm for this society and probably the question is not do we have something that needs to be worked out from our childhood? The appropriate question probably is, what do we have to work on from the experiences of our childhood?

The amazing thing about the human adventure is that no matter how horrendously awful our childhood was, as we work through it, we always find some memories of moments of happiness that had long since been forgotten. And no matter how perfect our family seemed on the surface, we always have some painful experiences to work through.

TRUE HAPPINESS **does not come from a perfect childhood. Happiness comes from claiming our unique childhood and working through the lessons it holds for us.**

❧ November 28

IN TOUCH WITH A POWER
GREATER THAN OURSELVES

It is not primarily abstract ideas which affect our spirituality, that is, our experience of and with God.

—Sandra M. Schneiders

We cannot approach God or the process of the universe through ideas. Theology is trying to think about God and often asks us to deny our *experience* of a power greater than ourselves.

When we learn to trust our own perceptions and experience, we discover that we begin to have a living relationship with the process of the universe. In fact, as we do our recovery work, we discover that when we are living out of our own process, we are one with the universe. We are not only in the holomovement, we *are* the holomovement.

This living process that is us is, at the same time, greater than ourselves. When we are truly ourselves, we are more than ourselves. We do not have to look for spirituality. We *are* spirituality. Spirituality permeates our being and all we are.

MY EXPERIENCE of the infinite cannot begin with my head and it includes all that I am. There's some relief in this knowing.

LAUGHTER

One loses many laughs by not laughing at oneself.
                              —Sara Jeannette Duncan

Well said! Part of the recovery process is to be able to
see how really funny we are in our disease. We need to
be able to see how really funny we are.

One of my better moments was when I was invited
to be the guest speaker at an important luncheon for
one of the Fortune 500 corporations. I had been out
camping just prior to this speaking engagement, so I
felt a little seedy. In order to make the right impression, I had brought a conservative business suit, silk
blouse, high-heeled boots, and panty hose. After being
in the wilderness for some time, I wasn't even sure I
knew how to get into this garb. Just before it was time
to speak, I went to the bathroom to "pee my anxieties
down the toilet" as we say in clinical circles. I came out
of the bathroom feeling a little cocky and ready to go.
Just as I reached the door to the auditorium, I was
aware of a breeze and realized that my skirt was caught
up in my panty hose and my rear was "exposed to the
Rockies." I had an instant opportunity for humility. Of
course it made a great opener for my speech.

WHEN WE SEE **how funny we are, we see how dear we are.**

GUILT

Women keep a special corner of their hearts for sins they have never committed.

—Cornelia Otis Skinner

We are so ready to take responsibility for everything that we are constantly feeling guilty.

If our spouse is feeling down or depressed it must be something we have done. If our children aren't doing well, it must be our fault. If the deadline isn't met, we should have put in more time. Women are so ready to take on the guilt of the world. It makes no difference whether we have committed these transgressions. If they exist, we must be responsible. Unfortunately, there are plenty of people around us who are happy to support us in these illusions of guilt.

We have never really stopped to see how self-centered it is to take on the responsibility for everything that happens, whether we are involved or not. When we take on the guilt for everything that happens around us, we make ourselves the center of everything.

THERE MUST be an easier way to be included.

❧ December 1

FINANCIAL SECURITY

Actually we are slaves to the cost of living.
                                    —Carolina Marin deJesus

All of us have to cope with the cost of living. Existing gets more and more expensive, and living seems sometimes as if it is only for the wealthy.

We have lost track of the difference between what we want and what we need. Everything has become a need. If we don't have what we think we need, it lowers our self-esteem and our feelings of worth. We can hardly remember what is important anymore.

We are important. Our children are important. Our relationships are important. The planet is important. Our lives are important.

LEST WE FORGET what we are all about, let's stop today to try to distinguish between need and want and remember.

INTERESTS/OVEREXTENDED

> *I am involved in so many things—both purely practical and also where my feelings, my life itself are concerned—possibly by my own fault or perhaps quite by chance, that it is going to take all my strength if I am going to get through them or over them.*

> —Isak Dinesen

Sometimes women who do too much get confused between healthy excitement about our work, a passion for our work, and workaholism. Passion moves to workaholism when it becomes destructive to the self and others. Workaholism isn't pursuing our interests. Workaholism doesn't give us time for our interests.

We often may overextend ourselves in the pursuit of our interests and the workaholic doesn't know when to stop. She just piles on more and more. The woman who has a healthy relationship with her interests is able to give her interests the time they deserve and savor them.

MY INTERESTS **add richness to my life, but not when I go after them compulsively.**

✤ December 3

FREEDOM

> *We must get in touch with our own liberating ludicrousness and practice being harmlessly deviant.*
>   —Sarah J. McCarthy

Freedom for me means being who I am. Professional women are supposed to have short, neat hair. I have long hair that has a mind of its own. It's harmless . . . and it's me. It is, indeed, liberating to be "ludicrous" and harmlessly deviant.

I once was a speaker at a university and while on campus was invited to attend a luncheon for the women faculty and staff on campus. During my luncheon speech, I asked if there was a dress code. I was quickly assured that the students could wear whatever they wanted. I told them I was asking about the women who worked on campus. They were all dressed exactly alike—suits, shirts, and some form of little tie. The only deviant was one woman who had a ruffle on her shirt!

FREEDOM is choosing the clothing that fits our personalities and feels good on us. This is one way we express who we are.

❧ December 4

THE GIFT OF OWNING MY PART

We cannot find peace if we are afraid of the windstorms of life.

—Elisabeth Kübler-Ross

Our lives don't always go smoothly. In fact, many of us have had many traumas and struggles. When we are in the midst of a difficult time, it is hard to see it as a gift. Nevertheless, at some megalevel, every experience is an opportunity for learning.

When we spend our energy blaming and complaining, we are handing over our power to those whom we blame. Our time and energy is well spent when we stop to say, "What is my part in this situation, and what do I have to learn from it?" In doing this, we are not blaming ourselves. We are not blaming at all. We are opening ourselves to glean whatever learnings are there for us. It is in this process that we become whole.

POWER OVER others does us no good at all. Owning my own part is the most effective method of recapturing my personal power that is known to me as a human.

✻ December 5

BEING IN CHARGE

Our strength is often composed of the weakness we're damned if we're going to show.

—Mignon McLaughlin

How in the world did I get to be in charge? There must be some mistake. I don't know what to do with this contract. I don't know how to raise these kids. I must have misrepresented myself for "them" to believe that I knew what I was doing. I am secretly at my best when someone else has the ultimate responsibility. Who has made this terrible mistake?

Often we truly believe that there must be someone who really has it all together and knows just what to do in every situation. Where is that person anyway? Maybe we can ask the right questions and get the right information, and then no one will suspect our charade.

YOU'RE IT, HONEY. Go for it.

❧ December 6

PATIENCE

That I did not fail was due in part to patience. . . .
                                        —Jane Goodall

Patience—*patience*. The word sounds vaguely familiar. It almost seems like one of those old-fashioned words that may drop out of the English language from disuse except in literary circles. Patience just is not a word in common usage these days.

Yet, in this age of instant everything, it just may be the practice of patience that saves our lives or at least prevents our failures.

I was born an Aries. Aries are great initiators. We are fantastic at generating a million creative new ideas a minute and flying around getting impossible tasks accomplished. For many years, I used my Aries status as a justification for my "inherent" lack of patience. I was just not "a constitutionally patient person."

Then, I began to see the limitations of impatience and lack of patience (the two being distinctly different in execution!). I began to see that lack of patience was my problem. It was not constitutional; patience could be learned, and was so delightful when practiced. My life has been so much easier with the practice of patience.

NOT EVERYTHING can be done "at once." In fact, the important things take time to percolate.

❧December 7

CLIMBING THE LADDER

The best career advice to give the young is, find out what you like doing best and get someone to pay you for doing it.

—Katherine Whilehaen

What we love doing often has no connection with our career choice. We live in a culture that teaches us to orient ourselves to what will sell. We have learned to ignore what we love and turn ourselves into a commodity. Commodities can be bought and sold, and we fear that we can be bought and sold. We don't feel that we have the luxury to see what it is we really want to be doing and even get paid for it.

We forget one very central and essential factor: if we are doing what we love, we will probably do it exceedingly well.

IF WE FOCUS on success, we will probably forget about living. If we focus on living and doing what we love, we have a good chance of being successful.

December 8

TEACHERS

If you can't be a good example, then you have to be a horrible warning.

—Catherine Aud

Some of our best teachers are those who have been a "horrible warning" for us. All too often, these people have not been easy for us to be around or have caused pain for us.

I recently was in a situation in which a group of people behaved not only inappropriately for the situation (it was a funeral) but actually rudely. Since I had a leadership responsibility, my first impulse, after I recovered from being stunned, was to jump up and stop them from upsetting the family. Then I realized that to cause an even bigger scene would be even more of a problem for everyone. When the bereaved family looked to me for guidance, I motioned for them to just let it pass, which it did quickly, and then proceeded as planned. In that situation, that group of people was a horrible warning for me. I did not want to be like them. They were teachers. Important teachers.

WE NEVER KNOW when and how our teachers will appear. Let's just hope we are ready for them.

❧ December 9

THINGS THAT HEARTEN

I see things every day that hearten me.

—Katie Couric

What a warm, positive statement. We don't need to focus on the negative. We don't need to put on our blinders. We can be ready to see those things that hearten us all around us. Just as beauty is in the eye of the beholder, so is ugly in the eye of the beholder. It is the eye that sees, and we have a lot of say about what the eye sees.

What if we begin to look at the world around us to try to see what heartens us? When we see the nail in our tire, what if we see the tire that still has some air in it? If we see the rain, what if we see the grass getting watered?

When we look at our children, what if we focus on the beauty in their eyes and not on the dirt on their face?

When we look at the piles on our desk, what if we focus on the piles that we have completed?

IN SEEING **what heartens us, we do, indeed, create our own reality.**

❧ December 10

FEELING TRAPPED

> *Women are the slave class that maintains the species in order to free the other half for the business of the world.*
> —Shulamith Firestone

We wanted to become professional women partly because we wanted to remove ourselves from being the "slave class that maintains the species." Yet, it is difficult fully to escape that trap. We find that any job can become a trap, whether we are full-time homemakers, volunteers, support personnel, or executive-level managers. Our society is set up in such a way that it takes a great many to support the work of a few. And even if we are part of the few, we are not always free.

We need to recognize that all of us, regardless of what we do, are part of the "business of the world," and the world needs all of us.

ACCEPTING who I am and what I have to offer is empowering to me and the society.

❧ December 11

EXPECTATIONS

Know that if you have a kind of cultured know-it-all in yourself who takes pleasure in pointing out what is not good, in discriminating, reasoning, and comparing, you are bound under a knave. I wish you could be delivered.

— Brenda Ueland

We don't need anyone else to criticize us. We have so many superhuman expectations of ourselves that the expectations of others pale into insignificance. We really believe that we should be able to handle everything. We really believe we should know everything. We really believe that we should be on top of everything. When we are caught unprepared, instead of just admitting it, we either get defensive or feel guilty (or both). It rarely occurs to us just to admit we are unprepared. We feel we should always be prepared for anything. (No control issues here!)

OUR EXPECTATIONS **keep us from crying "uncle" (or for any other relative help, for that matter).**

❧ December 12

SISSIES

Old age ain't no place for sissies.

—Bette Davis

Neither is any other age for that matter!

We women who do too much can hardly be accused of being sissies. In fact, we may be accused of being tough. Look at how much we do. Look how many things we can juggle. Look at how much we can handle. We're no sissies, so we should be well prepared for old age . . . or will we be?

Are we sissies about asking for what we need?

Are we sissies about taking time for ourselves even when there is so much to do?

Are we sissies about saying no?

Are we sissies about standing up for our beliefs even if no one else sees the world the same way we do?

Are we sissies about saying *enough?*

JUST BECAUSE we do too much doesn't eliminate us from being sissies.

❧ December 13

BECOMING

One is not born a woman, one becomes one.
                              —Simone de Beauvoir

We live in a society that puts so much emphasis upon youth, looks, and attractiveness that we have very few models for womanliness.

Without knowing how to get there, we are suddenly expected to be women and to have the wisdom and stature of a woman.

In a society that knows little about process, there is an assumption that one is a little girl and then suddenly one is a woman. In our sexualized culture, becoming a woman almost always is linked to our sexuality. Womanhood is much more than being sexual and producing babies. Womanhood is the progressive process of bringing all we have to offer as persons to ourselves and those around us.

I AM being a woman. That is a process, not a state.

❧December 14

STRENGTH

From a timid, shy girl I had become a woman of resolute character, who could no longer be frightened by the struggle with troubles.

—Anna Dostoevsky

Finding and accepting our strength is a very important aspect of knowing ourselves as women. Adolescents do not usually know their own strength, but women do. When we deny our strength, we give up pieces of who *we* are. When we use our strength for power over others, we deny who *they* are. Either way, we lose.

Much of our strength comes from knowing and accepting ourselves and accepting that we are not the center of the universe. As we accept ourselves, we come to realize that our strength is directly connected with and one with a power greater than ourselves. When we tap into that power, we know that we have all the strength we need for whatever comes.

AS THE OLD Ethiopian proverb states, "When spider webs unite, they can tie up a lion."

❧ December 15

SELF-CONFIDENCE

Class is an aura of confidence that is being sure without being cocky. Class has nothing to do with money. Class never runs scared. It is self-discipline and self-knowledge. It's the sure-footedness that comes with having proved you can meet life.

—Ann Landers

Self-confidence is so relaxing. There is no strain or stress when one is self-confident. Our lack of self-confidence mostly comes from trying to be someone we aren't. No wonder we do not feel confident when we are living a lie. When we realize that the best we have to bring to any situation is being just who we are, we relax. People who are cocky often show an alarming lack of self-confidence. They don't know what they have to offer. When we know what we have to offer and we bring it to each situation, that's all we need to do.

I LIKE being a classy woman. No show . . . no blow . . . just the facts.

❧ December 16

HOLIDAYS/FRANTIC

Holidays and frantic aren't necessarily synonymous.
—Anne Wilson Schaef

We see the holiday season coming and we immediately feel exhausted and overwhelmed. We have to maintain our usual workday and in addition, shop for gifts, decorate the house, do the extra holiday baking, attend additional social functions, and look great. For some of us, "the season to be jolly," becomes the season to wipe ourselves out. As women who do too much, we have come to dread the holiday season.

This is a good year for us to stop, take stock, and see what is really important for us this season. Perhaps we love the traditions. Which ones can we continue and be healthy? Perhaps we can try asking for help and stop trying to do everything ourselves. This season we have the opportunity to let ourselves feel the meaning of peace—peace within and peace with the world.

DOING THE HOLIDAY SEASON sanely is part of my healing process. I have that opportunity this season. Ho ho ho.

✤ December 17

HEALING

I will tell you what I have learned myself. For me, a long five- or six-mile walk helps. And one must go alone and every day.

— Brenda Ueland

Healing takes time. Healing is an everyday affair. Some traumatic events in our lives require physical, emotional, and/or spiritual healing, and sometimes we just need to let the nicks, chips, and dents from everyday living heal. Doing the work we do and holding things together the way we do takes its toll.

When we need these healing times, there is nothing better than a good long walk. It is amazing how the rhythmic movements of the feet and legs are so intimately attached to cobweb cleaners in the brain. And we must take a *long* walk, because at first we think about our problems. These thoughts dissipate over time, thus allowing the healing to begin and we are less focused on our thinking.

WHEN MY HEELS touch the earth, I am healing my wounds.

❧ December 18

LOVE

We can only learn to love by loving.

—Doris Murdock

Many women who do too much believe that there are tricks to loving. If we can just look sexy enough, we can make others love us. Or if we just take care of others and make ourselves indispensable, they will love us. We don't learn to love by loving, we try to control love by manipulation. Unfortunately, these methods do not teach us much about loving.

Loving is a risk. It is letting go of expectations and just allowing. Some of us doubt our capacity to love because we have been raised in dysfunctional families and never really have had much experience of clear loving. Loving always had strings attached or demands that we had to meet. Hence we have practiced loving as we learned it in our families.

Fortunately, we are capable of new learning. And it starts right inside of us. When we experience loving ourselves, we begin to learn by loving.

AS I LOVE MYSELF, it is only a short step to the loving of others.

❧ December 19

COMMUNICATION

If you have anything to tell me of importance, for God's sake begin at the end.

—Sara Jeannette Duncan

Women have always believed that the goal of communication is to bridge, connect, clarify, and facilitate understanding. We have often developed this skill and been good communicators.

Then we find that in our worklives, communication is used in quite different ways than we had realized. Communication is used to manipulate, control, confuse, and intimidate—to create barriers rather than to bridge them. Success is intimately linked with this confusing and confounding form of communication. We are told that we have to play the game.

Later we find that the people we admire often are very direct and refuse to play the game. We have been tempted to abandon our communication skills, and we sorely need them.

BEGINNING **at the end may be a good start. At least it's more direct.**

✤ December 20

Surely the strange beauty of the world must somewhere rest on pure joy!

—Louise Bogan

Indeed, the world is so beautiful . . . and so imaginative. Who would have thought to design a tree such that its limbs, when they become too heavy, send down another trunk, so that a single tree repeating this process many times over can eventually cover an area the size of an entire block? Imagine a tree that is so tall that we can't really see the top—a tree that has developed at least three methods of reproducing itself so as not to become extinct. Indeed, "the strange beauty of the world must somewhere rest on pure joy." We have the opportunity to experience that joy. When we notice, the strange beauty of the earth is all around us.

IT PROBABLY WON'T HURT to give thanks that the design and creation of the world was not left in our hands.

❧ December 21

INSPIRATION

Inspiration comes very slowly and quietly.
—Brenda Ueland

Sometimes we forget that to do our work well, whatever it is, we must have inspiration. This is true for any work, no matter how menial it may seem. Inspiration is the gentle listening to the wisdom of our inner being.

Brenda Ueland said that it comes slowly and quietly. I might also add that it comes when it wishes and not on demand. Like any process, we cannot force it. We must wait with it.

How sad that we have relegated inspiration to poets, artists, and writers! How sad that we cannot see that good child rearing requires inspiration, that good management requires inspiration, regardless of the task. When we take away the possibility of our own inspiration, we relegate ourselves to a tedious existence. Inspiration adds spice and zest to our lives and allows them to be lives, not existences.

WHEN I WAIT with inspiration, my time is not wasted.

CHOICES/FEAR/CHANGE

> *Change really becomes a necessity when we try not to do it.*
> —Anne Wilson Schaef

Risk and fear—we will do anything to avoid them both. Where did we get the idea that it is bad to feel fear and that we cannot handle our fear? We will do anything to avoid the fear of making a choice. We have another baby, or take on more work, or get busy with a new project around the house—anything.

We have so much fear of facing ourselves and confronting the choices we need to make that we are willing to wreck our lives and the lives of those around us in order not to have to make a choice.

We always resent it when others make decisions for us, *and* we do not want to be responsible for our choices. If we can manage to get someone else to make a choice for us, then we do not have to own the consequences.

I SAY I WANT to be my own person, and sometimes that scares me to death. . . . That's OK.

❧ December 23

> *If you see a whole thing, it seems that it's always beautiful. Planets. Lives. But close up a world's all dirt and rocks. And day to day, life's a hard job, you get tired, you lose the pattern.*
>
> —Ursula K. Le Guin

In doing too much, being stressed, and feeling tired, we often become embedded in the small details. It seems like we do everything we have to do—all the little things—and that's our life. Life is hard. When it becomes hard, we lose the pattern. We lose the picture of the whole and it doesn't seem beautiful at all. It's all rocks and dirt.

Maybe this is what gives God the edge on us. God can always see the bigger picture and how beautiful we really are.

We can see the bigger picture, too. We can see that our children are beautiful beings as well as tasks. We can see that each little thing we do has significance. We can see that everything, but everything, is much larger than it appears and is part of a whole.

WHEN WE LOSE perspective and pattern, we lose the beauty in our lives and the whole.

❧ December 24

CAUSES/DUALISM

> *The main dangers in this life are the people who want to change everything . . . or nothing.*
>
> —Lady Astor

How aptly put! Lady Astor put her finger on the meaning of dualism and the horror of being caught in a dualism. Those who want to change everything often become ruthless in their laser focus upon what they know is right.

Those who want to change nothing have become so enured to themselves and other beings that they only pass through life not looking to the right or to the left. Neither group does much for itself or anyone else. Actually, both groups operate out of the same self-centered focus.

What is the third option? The third option is to be present to ourselves and others, accepting those things which we cannot change, changing the things we can, and knowing the difference.

WHEN I get caught up in a "cause," I become the problem. When I do nothing about the world in which I live, I am the problem.

❧ December 25

CONNECTEDNESS

God knows no distance.

—Charleszetta Waddles

How far away we seem at times from any Higher Power. We simply cannot connect with a power greater than ourselves, and we lose faith in its existence.

It is important to remember that the distance is within *us*. We are the ones who have moved away from that power and that connectedness. It has not moved away from us.

Our rushing around, our busyness, our constant caretaking and compulsive working leave little or no time or energy for anyone or anything to enter. Yet when we stop to notice, the connection with this power greater than ourselves is always there. It has never left us. *We* have left us.

THE DISTANCE is mine. The potential for connectedness is mine, also.

❧ December 26

GROWTH

> *Lying, walking, sitting in this room, she felt herself ripening and coloring.*
>
> —Meridel LeSueur

We have such a cult of youth in this society that, for a woman, growing older is a terrifying experience. Meridel LeSueur's usage of the words "ripening" and "coloring" are very soothing. If I see myself ripening and becoming richer as I grow older, if I see myself developing a more intricate patina, my process of growth takes on a different tone.

We have two big dogs in our household, a seven-year-old Great Dane queen (seven is old for a Great Dane!) and a happy tramp–like German shepherd about two years old. Although she is busy being a queen, and he is busy growing up, they have the most beautiful, devoted, and caring relationship. He does not seem to mind that she is an "old lady" and has some grey hair. As I watch them, I realize that human beings are probably the only species that worship youth and disdain maturity. Among animals, it just doesn't seem to matter.

I COULD NOT KNOW what I know today if I weren't the age I am. I have the continual opportunity to grow. And age adds patina.

SIGNIFICANCE

> *The key to realizing a dream is to focus not on success but on significance—and then even the small steps and little victories along your path will have greater meaning.*
>
> —Oprah Winfrey

What in the world ever made you think that your small steps, the little things you do, are not significant? What a hoot!

When I am told to take one step at a time, I always have a little inner giggle. Have you ever tried to take two steps at a time? Doesn't work.

We have to content ourselves in the knowledge that everything that we do is significant. Many years ago, one of the exercises that Virginia Satir used to do to teach this was to tie a family up with one single rope. In no time they experienced that every little movement affected everyone else in the family.

And so it is in life—nothing, but nothing—we do is insignificant. Everything we do affects someone else and has much, much more meaning than we may realize at that moment. We live in an interconnected universe. We may not like to recognize the responsibility of knowing that everything we do has significance. And, it does.

JUST BECAUSE we have been taught that we and what we do are insignificant doesn't mean it's true.

❧ December 28

CLARITY/CHANGES/GROWTH

*Then I began to realize that I had to take another step in
my evolution and growth.*

—Eileen Caddy

We sometimes avoid getting clear because we intuitively know that when we get clear we will have to make some changes in our lives. We are so accustomed to doing what is expected of us that it is difficult to know what we want or need. We can so easily give in to the demands of others, especially if they are in positions of authority, that we find ourselves confused and lacking clarity.

In spite of our confusion, our inner process continues to push us toward our evolution and growth. Something in us struggles for clarity. Yet, with clarity comes another step.

Judith K. Knowlton said, "When I keep putting something off, it may not be procrastination, but a decision I've already made and not yet admitted to myself."

Will our clarity push us toward acting on that decision?

How good are we at avoiding clarity and decisions we have already made?

GROWTH **and evolution are like breathing and eating . . .
natural and intimately part of being human.**

❧December 29

LETTING OUR LIVES HAPPEN

Fate keeps happening.

—Anita Loos

Our lives are not set in stone. Lives, like flowers, continue to unfold. We have options and we have choices all along the way.

Certainly we have been influenced by our past and the many forces that have impinged upon us in our formative years. Yet we do have the ability to alter our present and our future.

Fate is a process that continues to emerge. As we accept who we are, we have the possibility of becoming someone else. That is the paradox of life and of living.

When I can let life happen, I feel better. When I can participate in the happening of my life, I soar.

LIFE IS **in the living. The process of life keeps happening.**

❧ December 30

COMPASSION/LOVING

Nobody has ever measured, even poets, how much the heart can hold.

—Zelda Fitzgerald

Some of us have become estranged from our feelings of compassion and love. We have believed that we had to become so tough and that we had to keep so busy that love and compassion became luxuries we could ill afford. Surely we could maintain our humanness with a few tax-deductible checks to the proper charities at the end of the year!

Yet, we know down deep that we are loving, compassionate women. When we give ourselves time, we care about people, and there are many things we love about our lives. Our hearts have a limitless capacity for caring and compassion.

TO LET MY HEART swell with feelings of love and compassion is better than any combination of vitamins and exercise I could ever devise.

❧ December 31

BEAUTY

Happily may I walk.
May it be beautiful before me.
May it be beautiful behind me.
May it be beautiful below me.
May it be beautiful above me.
May it be beautiful all around me.
In beauty it is finished.

—Navajo prayer

If one reads this prayer very slowly, one feels its immensely profound simplicity. Imagine ourselves surrounded by beauty! When we think of being surrounded by beauty, we think of some island paradise or Shangri-la.

Yet, when we read this poem slowly, we begin to realize that we *are* surrounded by beauty! We see that this prayer is not only a request, it is simultaneously a statement of fact.

My life does have elements of beauty before, behind, below, and above me. I am surrounded by beauty.

WHEN I END my year in beauty, I am ready for whatever comes.

❧ Alternate Meditation 1

CREATIVITY/ALONE TIME

I can always be distracted by love, but eventually I get horny for my creativity.

— Gilda Radner

Nothing can replace creativity in our lives—not work, not love, not children, nothing. We may be creative in all these areas, Yet our creative impulses must find their own avenue for expression.

Regardless of how interesting and challenging our work is and how creative we are with our work, we need times of quiet reflection to tap into the deep recesses of our being and see what is perking there. There is no substitute for our creativity, which is usually tapped when we are alone.

I LIKE the way Gilda Radner puts it: "eventually I get horny for my creativity."

❧ Alternate Meditation 2

DOING OUR WORK

The household is not only a home, but a source of lucrative careers.

—Linda F. Radke

Ms. Radke writes about household careers—nannies, maids, butlers, and so forth. Lots of careers can go on in the home.

When I saw her statement, I thought about some of the writing I had done about dysfunctional companies and organizations. Functional people don't do well in dysfunctional organizations. As we get healthier, we don't "fit" so well. We get pressured to get back in line and be dysfunctional like everyone else. Many of us become isolated or decide that it is time to leave, take a risk with our own entrepreneurial efforts.

So many women are setting up their own businesses creatively and successfully. So many are seeing that we don't have to be like water and seek our lowest level.

WHATEVER IT IS we want to do with our work lives, we need to let ourselves know. There is always room for innovators and entrepreneurs.

❧ Alternate Meditation 3

PERFECTIONISM/PROCRASTINATION

I know if I do it just one more time, I can get it right.

—Anonymous

And one more time, and one more time, and one more time. Perfectionism is a difficult and impossible taskmaster. Also, perfectionism is a way of defining the task and ourselves from outside and may have nothing to do with what the task really is or who we really are.

In fact, we may use perfectionism to keep ourselves from getting anything done. If it has to be done perfectly, why even start? Perfectionism and procrastination go hand in hand, and accomplish nothing.

We need to remember that we are doing the task at hand and therefore what we have to bring to the task is ourselves, our accumulated knowledge and experience, and our creativity. Who could ask for anything more?

LET ME NOT ASK **for anything more today than to bring what I have to each task at hand.**

✺ Alternate Meditation 4

NOURISHING OURSELVES

When you recover or discover something that nourishes your soul and brings joy, care enough about yourself to make room for it in your life.

—Jean Shinoda Bolen

When we are constantly rushing around and busy, we are in special need of nourishment (that isn't bad for us and doesn't put on weight!). When we are moving so fast, all too often we have difficulty glimpsing those things that are nourishing to us as we speed by. It's like all those car ads on TV where the cars are careening and flying through absolutely gorgeous landscapes. Do you suppose they are noticing the landscape? I hope not, for at that speed, it could be very dangerous to take your eyes off the road (our lives are a bit like that, aren't they?).

Yet, there are things that nourish us—a massage, a pedicure, rose-scented spray, fresh flowers, a favorite movie, a secret place, a good book. The list is endless.

LET'S SEE if we can care enough about ourselves to make room in our lives for those things that nourish us.

❦ Alternate Meditation 5

TRUST

> *Believing in our hearts that who we are is enough is the*
> *key to a more satisfying and balanced life.*
>
> —Ellen Sue Stern

I am enough! I have always been afraid of being too much or too little. What a relief I feel when I just sit with the possibility that I am enough. Can it really be true that I am not what I do or what I produce or what I accomplish? What if I am enough and I accomplish what I want to do? Would that truly be enough? Probably!

I would like a "satisfying and balanced" life. I would like more time and energy for my work, myself, and those I love. When I recognize that *I am enough,* I will have what I want and need.

I WILL SIT **with this feeling of being enough and let it be with me today.**

✺ Alternate Meditation 6

RELATIONSHIPS

> *Girls must be encouraged to go on [after college], to make a life plan. It has been shown that girls with this kind of commitment are less eager to rush into early marriage. . . . Most of them marry, of course, but on a much more mature basis. Their marriages then are not an escape but a commitment shared by two people that become part of their commitment to themselves and society.*

> —Betty Friedan

We don't know much about healthy relationships in this society. Too often we look to relationships as an external fix. We expect them to give us our identity and make our lives all right. When we do this, we bring no one to the relationship. We are like jello, and we ask our partners to give us form by means of a relationship. Without the external mold of a relationship, the jello dissolves into a puddle. Who wants to or even can relate to a puddle of jello?

IF I WANT to be in a relationship, I have to bring someone to it . . . me.

❧ Alternate Meditation 7

BEING TORN/GUILT

No woman should be shamefaced in attempting, through her work, to give back to the world a portion of its heart.

—Louise Bogan

It is difficult for women to do our own work. Women artists are frequently expected to keep house, run a family, do the carpool, cook all the meals, do the cleaning, and be able to spend their "spare" moments in their (usually makeshift) studio with their work. Life is never easy for an artist in this culture. Life is almost impossible for a woman artist in this culture.

And women artists are not alone in this struggle. Any woman who does too much cannot help but see the effect of overworking. Any woman who does too much cannot help but see the effect of her addiction on her family. Even when we firmly believe that our work should come first, we feel terrible pangs of guilt when our spouses and children have to make appointments with us to see us at all.

Yet, we all want to give back to the world a portion of its heart. Perhaps it can be through our children or through what we produce.

A WORKING WOMAN is one of the best balancing acts in this three-ring circus we call life. At least we are not alone in struggling with this issue.

✄ Alternate Meditation 8

CREATIVITY

*They say the moon is feminine. What will happen to me
if I bathe myself in the creative feminine?*

—Michelle

I like the image of the moonlight acting as an activator to help the emergence of what is already there within me!

If I bathe myself in moonlight, what miraculous and surprising images might emerge?

I suppose the real issue is not the magic of the moonlight, but whether I am willing to slow down enough to let any form of nature have an opportunity to bathe me.

Ancient peoples knew that connecting with nature released curative and creative energies. I, too, need nature in my life.

GETTING in nature may not be easy and even cities have moonlight.

❧ Alternate Meditation 9

HAVING HELP

I am where I am because of the bridges I crossed. Sojourner Truth was a bridge. Harriet Tubman was a bridge. Ida B. Wells was a bridge. Madame C. J. Walker was a bridge. Fannie Lou Hamer was a bridge.

—Oprah Winfrey

Whatever we have made of our lives, we have never done it alone.

First, we have our ancestors to thank. Quite literally, we would not be here if it weren't for them. If they had not lived we would not live. (Did you ever stop to think about that?)

Then, we have our DNA, which carries in it probably much more than we realize. Many scholars believe our DNA carries not only our physical characteristics but our memories and learnings.

Then, we have the women who went before us, who courageously paved the way and fought the battles so that our lives as women would perhaps be a little better.

WE HAVE HAD to make our lives ourselves, and we have not had to do it alone.

❧ Alternate Meditation 10

CREATIVITY

Why should we all use our creative power . . . ? Because there is nothing that makes people so generous, joyful, lively, bold and compassionate, so indifferent to fighting and the accumulation of objects and money.

—Brenda Ueland

So much of our frustration and irritability is a reaction to not using our creative powers. All of us have areas of creativity, and each of us has a unique creativity that is especially related to our talents and personality. Whenever we look at others and think, "I can't paint like that," or "I don't have the talent she does," we move a step further away from realizing what *we* have.

When we block our creativity, we lose touch with our joy and our liveliness. Is it any wonder that we become cantankerous and try to fill up the loneliness for our creative selves with money and things—which never quite do the job.

WHAT I REALLY search for is me, and I am by nature creative.

✌ Alternate Meditation 11

HOUSEWORK

Cleaning your house while your kids are still growing is like shoveling the walk before it stops snowing.

—Phyllis Diller

I never understand why housework is not added to the list of inevitables like taxes and death. No matter what we are trying to get done or how much we need a rest, etc., housework is always calling to us like the siren's song: "Come do me . . . come do me." I have thought of inventing a birth control spray that prevents the housework from reproducing itself while we sleep. When we get up in the morning there always seems to be more housework than when we went to bed.

The nice thing about housework, of course, is that it doesn't go away. We can go ahead and do some of our creative work or soak in the tub, and it will be there waiting when we come back to it.

SINCE HOUSEWORK is always there waiting for me, I might as well go ahead and do what I want.

❧ Alternate Meditation 12

ACTION/CONTROL

I have always had a dread of becoming a passenger in life.

—Princess Margrethe of Denmark

As women, we have been raised to expect someone to take care of us. Most professional women prize our independence. Yet down deep we often have a secret wish that someone else would take responsibility for our lives. Frequently we vacillate between wishing to be passengers in life and asserting that we can handle things ourselves. Sometimes we get stuck between these two polarities. We believe that we must either resign ourselves to going along for the ride or we must be in the engine running the train. We do not see the third option—take responsibility for our lives and simultaneously turn them over to a power greater than ourselves.

To participate in our lives does not mean that we control our lives. Not to control our lives does not mean that we are passive.

I DO NOT NEED to choose between being a passenger or being an engineer. I can live my process.

❧ Alternate Meditation 13

HONESTY/HONORING ONESELF

> *How many are silenced, how many women never "find their voice" because in order to get to their art they would have to scream?*
>
> —Ann Clark

Some of us find the words "obligations to myself" foreign. We have been raised to believe that we should sacrifice ourselves in order to be good. Then others of us have reacted to the female cult of self-sacrifice and decided that we needed to be selfish and to focus upon ourselves. Often we bounce back and forth between these two choices. Unfortunately (or fortunately, as the case may be), neither is satisfactory. Either way, we feel lonely, at loose ends, and unfulfilled.

The third option is to *honor* ourselves. When we honor ourselves and give out of that honoring, our giving is very clean. If we are not honoring ourselves, our giving has strings attached and is uncomfortable for the giver and the receiver.

WHEN I HONOR myself, I discover the magic of my voice and my productions.

❧ Alternate Meditation 14

FREEDOM

Freedom means choosing your burden.

—Hephzibah Menuhin

No one has complete freedom. Complete freedom is a myth that is terrifying to most and a dream-filled illusion for others. While we are wrestling with our terror of complete freedom or fighting the constrictions in our lives, we forget the freedoms we already have. We have the freedom to choose our burdens.

Women who have no children have chosen the burden of full-time work *without* the freedom that relating to children brings. Women who have chosen to have children have chosen the burden of rearing children (and often full-time work out of the home also!). Whatever our choices, we have made them. They are ours. We have the freedom to live with them.

I HAVE CHOSEN my burdens. Sometimes I don't see the freedom in that.

❧ Index

Acceptance - Feb. 11, Mar. 12, Mar. 17, Apr. 15, June 19, July 24, Oct. 23, Nov. 15, Nov. 18

Accomplishments-May 31

Achievement, need for-Jan. 8

Action-June 27, Nov. 8, Alternate Meditation 12

Adjusting-Apr. 19

Advice, giving-Apr. 17

Alone time-Feb. 3, Mar. 15, July 12, July 19, Aug. 31, Nov. 21, Alternate Meditation 1

Ambition-Sept. 8, Nov. 18

Amends-Feb. 20, Mar. 12, July 6

Amusing God-Jan. 16

Anger-Jan. 9, Mar. 14

Anguish-May 11

Animals-Jan. 26

Appreciation-Apr. 18, Nov. 20

Arrogance-May 23

Awareness-Mar. 18, May 17, Sept. 5, Oct. 18

Awe-Aug. 17, Oct. 17

Balance-July 16

Beauty-Apr. 28, June 11, Oct. 15, Oct. 17, Dec. 31

Becoming-Mar. 17, Mar. 30, Oct. 2, Dec. 13

Being direct-Oct. 22

Being in charge-June 5, July 13, Dec. 5

Being powerful-June 25

Being torn-July 14, Alternate Meditation 7

Belief-Jan. 14, Feb. 6, Apr. 25, June 6

Busyness-Mar. 25, Apr. 11, Apr. 26, May 9, May 28, Aug. 11, Aug. 15, Sept. 29

Causes-Nov. 1, Dec. 24

Celebrations-Aug. 28

Change-Jan. 11, Dec. 22, Dec. 28; becoming the- Sept. 23

Children-Oct. 16; raising-Aug. 26

Choices-Jan. 3, Feb. 24, Apr. 27, Sept. 27, Dec. 22

Clarity-Sept. 21, Dec. 28

Clutter-June 8
Commitment-Oct. 1
Common destinies-Aug. 5
Common sense-Jan. 2
Communication-Feb. 10, Oct. 28, Dec. 19
Compassion-Jan. 13, Dec. 30
Competition-Feb. 12
Confidence-July 23
Conflict-Feb. 11, May 21
Confusion-May 22, June 15, Sept. 22, Oct. 10
Connectedness-Apr. 5, May 22, Dec. 25
Contentment-June 10
Contradictions-July 30
Control-Jan. 5, Jan. 19, Jan. 20, Jan. 28, Feb. 17, Mar. 20, May 23,
    Aug. 25, Sept. 2, Sept. 5, Oct. 8, Oct. 13, Oct. 20, Nov. 10,
    Nov. 14, Alternate Meditation 12
Coping-Nov. 16
Courage-Mar. 26, May 2, June 24
Crazy, feeling-Feb. 15, Mar. 2, June 16, Oct. 3, Nov. 16
Creativity-Feb. 17, Oct. 27, Nov. 12, Alternate Meditation 1,
    Alternate Meditation 8, Alternate Meditation 10
Crisis-Jan. 5, Nov. 3
Crutches, avoiding-July 21
Curiosity-June 13
Cycles-July 23
Deadlines-Nov. 6
Decisions-Mar. 22
Demanding too much of oneself-Sept. 7
Depression-July 31
Despair-Mar. 19, Mar. 28, May 3, Oct. 9
Discouragement-Mar. 27
Distractibility-Apr. 11
Doing our work-Alternate Meditation 2
Doing the best we can-July 18
Doors-July 17
Dreams-May 24, Sept. 28, Oct. 25
Dualism-Dec. 24

Duty-Aug. 21
Enthusiasm-July 9
Excellence-Sept. 26
Excuses-Jan. 3
Exhaustion-Jan. 5, Feb. 5, May 28, June 3
Expectations-Feb. 14, June 20, Aug. 14, Dec. 11
Expendability-Jan. 28
Failure-Apr. 6
Fear-Jan. 21, Jan. 28, Mar. 26, Apr. 29, Sept. 30, Oct. 21, Dec. 22
Feelings-Feb. 11, Mar. 4, Mar. 20, Sept. 15; sharing-June 17
Fixers and Fixees-Nov. 4
Forgiveness-Mar. 21, May 30, July 6; of mistakes-Jan. 27
Frantic-Feb. 18, Dec. 16
Freedom-Mar. 4, June 1, Aug. 3, Oct. 4, Dec. 3
    Alternate Meditation 14
Frenzy-Jan. 1
Friendship-Apr. 8, July 7, Sept. 29
Fun-July 29
Genius-Aug. 8
Gifts-Jan. 15, Feb. 4, Apr. 1, Sept. 17; of owning my part-Dec. 4
Goals-Feb. 12, June 4, Aug. 10
Gratitude-Feb. 9, Mar. 24, Aug. 6; for having loved-May 29
Growth-July 8, Aug. 7, Dec. 26, Dec. 28
Guilt-Apr. 23, May 14, July 12, Sept. 18, Nov. 2, Nov. 30,
    Alternate Meditation 7
Hanging in there-Mar. 23, Nov. 9
Happiness-Feb. 2, June 30, July 31, Aug. 25, Nov. 27
Harmony-Aug. 5
Healing-May 25, Dec. 17
Hearten, things that-Dec. 9
Help, asking for-May 16, Aug. 16; having-Alternate Meditation 9
Higher Power-Mar. 1, Mar. 9, Sept. 3, Nov. 28
Holidays-Aug. 2, Dec. 16
Honesty-Jan. 23, Apr. 15, Sept. 1, Alternate Meditation 13
Honoring oneself-Alternate Meditation 13
Hopes-May 24, Oct. 25
Housekeeping-Mar. 11, Alternate Meditation 11

Humility-July 24
Humor-Jan. 4, July 3
Illusions-Jan. 6, Feb. 7
Impression management-Feb. 29, Aug. 29
Independence-Apr. 16
Indispensable-Oct. 8
Inner knowings-Aug. 18
Inspiration- Nov. 13, Dec. 21
Integrity-Apr. 4, Sept. 20
Interests-Dec. 2
Intergenerational patterns-Apr. 3
Interruptions-Aug. 30
Intimacy-Jan. 24, May 10, Aug. 12
Intuition-Nov. 7
Inventory-Apr. 20
Isolation-Apr. 30
Joyfulness-June 30, Aug. 1, Sept. 2, Dec. 20
Judgmentalism-Oct. 12
Just being-June 12
Keeping others down-June 2
Knowing when to let go-Oct. 19
Ladder, climbing the-Feb. 9, Dec. 7
Laughter-Feb. 28, Nov. 29
Learning-Sept. 4
Letting go-Feb. 23, Mar. 3, Nov. 10
Life: living fully-Apr. 2, May 26, June 13, June 26, July 2, Aug. 9,
    Sept. 13; ebb and flow-June 22; letting it happen-Dec. 29
Limits, reaching our-Sept. 12
Living in the now-Oct. 23
Loneliness-Mar. 5, May 9, May 22, July 27, Aug. 27
Love-May 12, Nov. 11, Dec. 18
Loving-Dec. 30
Man's world-Aug. 13
Manipulation-Apr. 29
Meanness-Mar. 31
Medications-Feb. 8
Men, relating to-May 19

Menopause-Jan. 12

Minds: monotone-Apr. 7, Oct. 11

Mirrors-Apr. 13

Mistakes-Mar. 12; forgiveness of-Jan. 27

Moment: being present to the: May 20, Sept. 19, Oct. 7;
    living in-Jan. 18,

Morality, personal-Feb. 13

Moving meditations-Oct. 5

Moving on-Aug. 20

Multi-Tasking-Jan. 30

My life-June 21

Myths-Feb. 7

Negativism-Jan. 10, Apr. 14, June 15

Neglect-July 20

Niceness-July 1

Nourishing ourselves-Alternate Meditation 4

Obsessed, being-Oct. 30

Obstacles-Jan. 22

Older, getting-Oct. 2

Oneness-Oct. 17, Oct. 29

Oneself: nurturing-Feb. 26

Organizational change-Oct. 26

Others, needing-Oct. 30

Overextended-Dec. 2

Overwhelmed, feeling-May 5, Sept. 14, Oct. 14

Pain-Feb. 25

Panic-Sept. 27

Parenting-May 13, Oct. 24

Passion-Mar. 29

Patience-Mar. 22, Dec. 6

Perfectionism-Feb. 27, July 27, Nov. 25,
    Alternate Meditation 3

Perspective-Dec. 23; losing-Jan. 25

Physical health-Apr. 10

Power-June 29

Powerlessness-Jan. 29

Present, living in the-May 4, June 18

Prisons-July 5
Process: awareness of-Feb. 17, May 27, June 14, Oct. 1, Oct. 20;
    in touch with-Mar. 1
Procrastination-Nov. 6, Alternate Meditation 3
Productivity-Feb. 7
Projects, juggling-Jan. 10, Feb. 19
Projectless: being-Apr. 24, Oct. 31
Promises, unrealistic-Mar. 19
Questions-July 15
Reality-Apr. 20, Aug. 16; admitting our-July 10
Recognition-Sept. 6
Regret-Mar. 11
Relationships-Mar. 6, Alternate Meditation 6;
    nurturing-Sept. 24
Resentments-Mar. 3
Responsibility-Feb. 24, May 14, July 19
Right on-Nov. 26
Rigidity-Jan. 7
Rushing-Jan. 1, Apr. 11
Ruthlessness-Jan. 13
Sadness-Aug. 20
Sanity-Mar. 7, Oct. 6
Secrets-Aug. 24
Security-Jan. 11; financial-Nov. 5, Dec. 1
Self: acceptance of-June 19, Sept. 6; giving away-Jan. 31;
    honoring-Sept. 27; unwrapping to us-May 7
Self-Affirmation-Mar. 8, June 29
Self-Awareness-Apr. 21, Nov. 17
Self-Confidence-Dec. 15
Self-Deception-Jan. 6
Self-Esteem-Mar. 9
Self-Respect-Apr. 22
Serenity-Mar. 10, May 8, Sept. 11
Shifting perceptions-June 7
Significance-Dec. 27
Sissies-Dec. 12
Sleep-May 28

Solitude-Feb. 22, Nov. 24
Solutions-June 9
Spiritual life-Mar. 13
Starting over-Sept. 10
Strength-Dec. 14
Struggle-Aug. 23
Stubbornness-Nov. 9
Success-Feb. 9, Apr. 4, July 22, Aug. 14
Support-Sept. 27
Taking our place-May 15
Talents-May 18
Teachers-Dec. 8
Tears-Mar. 16
Thank you-June 23
Thinking-Jan. 17; confused-Sept. 25, Oct. 12
Time-Feb. 16; management of-Nov. 19; unstructured-Apr. 12
Today-May 1
Toxic people-July 28
Trapped, feeling-Apr. 27, Dec. 10
Trust-July 26, Alternate Meditation 5
Truth-Aug. 4
Turning it over-Nov. 23
Understanding-July 4
Vacations-Aug. 2
Vague structure-Sept. 16
Values-Feb. 21
Victims-Apr. 9
Weekends-Apr. 12
What's next-July 11
Wholeness-June 28, Nov. 22, Dec. 23
Wisdom-June 14, Sept. 9
Women's perceptions-May 6
Wonder-July 25, Aug. 22
Work-Aug. 4, Sept. 30, Nov. 1;
    as a sacred possibility-Feb. 1
Worrying-Sept. 17
Youth-Aug. 19